TOP TRAILS™

Olympic National Park & Vicinity

MUST-DO HIKES FOR EVERYONE

Written by

Douglas Lorain

🐾 **WILDERNESS PRESS** . . . *on the trail since 1967*

Top Trails Olympic National Park & Vicinity: Must-Do Hikes for Everyone

First edition 2014
Copyright © 2014 by Douglas Lorain
Cover and interior photos, maps, and elevation profiles by Douglas Lorain
Cover design: Frances Baca Design and Scott McGrew
Text design: Frances Baca Design

ISBN: 978-0-89997-732-4; eISBN: 978-0-89997-733-1
Manufactured in the United States of America

Library of Congress Cataloging-in-Publication Data
Lorain, Douglas, 1962-
  Olympic National Park & vicinity : must-do hikes for everyone / written by Douglas
Lorain. — 1st edition.
     pages cm — (Top trails series)
  Includes bibliographical references and index.
  ISBN 978-0-89997-732-4 (alk. paper) — ISBN 0-89997-732-4 (alk. paper) — ISBN
978-0-89997-733-1 (eISBN)
  1. Hiking—Washington (State)—Olympic National Park—Guidebooks. 2. Hiking—
Washington (State)—Olympic National Park Region—Guidebooks. 3. Trails—
Washington (State)—Olympic National Park—Guidebooks. 4. Trails—Washington
(State)—Olympic National Park Region—Guidebooks. 5. Olympic National Park
(Wash.)—Guidebooks. 6. Olympic National Park Region (Wash.)—Guidebooks. I. Title.
  GV199.42.W22O495 2014
  796.5109795—dc23
                        2014015744

Published by: **Wilderness Press**
               c/o Keen Communications
               PO Box 43673
               Birmingham, AL 35243
               800-443-7227
               info@wildernesspress.com
               wildernesspress.com

Visit our website for a complete listing of our books and for ordering information.
Distributed by Publishers Group West
Cover photo: View west from upper reaches of Deer Ridge Trail (Trail 29)

SAFETY NOTICE: Although Keen Communications/Wilderness Press and the author
have made every attempt to ensure that the information in this book is accurate at press
time, they are not responsible for any loss, damage, injury, or inconvenience that may
occur to anyone while using this book. You are responsible for your own safety and health
while in the wilderness. The fact that a trail is described in this book does not mean that
it will be safe for you. Be aware that trail conditions can change from day to day. Always
check local conditions, know your own limitations, and consult a map and compass.

The Top Trails™ Series

Wilderness Press

When Wilderness Press published *Sierra North* in 1967, no other trail guide like it existed for the Sierra backcountry. The first run sold out in less than two months, and its success heralded the beginning of Wilderness Press. Since our founding, we have expanded our territories to cover California, Alaska, Hawaii, the US Southwest, the Pacific Northwest, New England, Canada, and the Southeast.

Wilderness Press continues to publish comprehensive, accurate, and readable outdoor books. Hikers, backpackers, kayakers, skiers, snowshoers, climbers, cyclists, and trail runners rely on Wilderness Press for accurate outdoor adventure information.

Top Trails

In its Top Trails guides, Wilderness Press has paid special attention to organization so that you can find the perfect hike each and every time. Whether you're looking for a steep trail to test yourself or a gentle walk in the park, a romantic waterfall or a lakeside view, Top Trails will lead you there.

Each Top Trails guide contains routes for everyone. The trails selected provide a sampling of the very best that the region has to offer. These are the must-do hikes with every feature of the area represented.

Every book in the Top Trails series offers:

- The Wilderness Press commitment to accuracy and reliability
- Ratings and rankings for each trail
- Distances and approximate times
- Easy-to-follow trail notes
- Map and permit information

Olympic National Park & Vicinity Trails

TRAIL NUMBER AND NAME	Page	Difficulty -1 2 3 4 5+	Length in Miles	Type	Day Hiking	Backpacking	Mountain Biking	Horses	Dogs Allowed	Child-Friendly
1. The Olympic Coast										
1 Cape Flattery	36	2	1.4	↗	🚶				🐕	👫
2 Shi Shi Beach and Point of the Arches	41	3	7.8	↗	🚶	🎒				
3 Ozette Triangle	47	3–4	9.0	↻	🚶	🎒				
4 Rialto Beach and Hole-in-the-Wall	55	2	3.0	↗	🚶				🐕	👫
5 Toleak Point	59	4	12.4	↗		🎒				
6 Jefferson Cove	66	3	5.2	↗	🚶					
7 Ruby Beach	71	1 and 3	5.8	↗	🚶					👫
2. West Region: The Rain Forests										
8 Hall of Mosses and Spruce Nature Trails	84	1	2.2	↻	🚶					👫
9 South Fork Hoh River Trail	90	2	4.7	↗	🚶	🎒				👫
10 Quinault Rain Forest Loop	96	2	4.0	↻	🚶				🐕	👫
11 Pony Bridge, Enchanted Valley, and Anderson Glacier	102	3–5	5.0–38.4	↗	🚶	🎒		🐴		
12 Colonel Bob	111	5	8.2	↗	🚶	🎒		🐴	🐕	
3. Northwest Region: Lake Crescent and Sol Duc Areas										
13 Mount Muller Loop	126	5	13.0	↻	🚶		🚲	🐴	🐕	
14 Sol Duc Falls–Lover's Lane Loop	133	2	5.9	↻	🚶					👫
15 High Divide Loop	140	5	20.3	↻		🎒		🐴		
16 Marymere Falls	152	1	1.6	↗	🚶					👫
17 Mount Storm King Viewpoint	156	3	3.2	↗	🚶					
18 Spruce Railroad Trail	161	2	5.8	↗	🚶		🚲	🐴	🐕	👫
19 The Cove and Salt Creek Country Park	166	2	2.2	↗	🚶				🐕	👫

TRAIL FEATURES TABLE

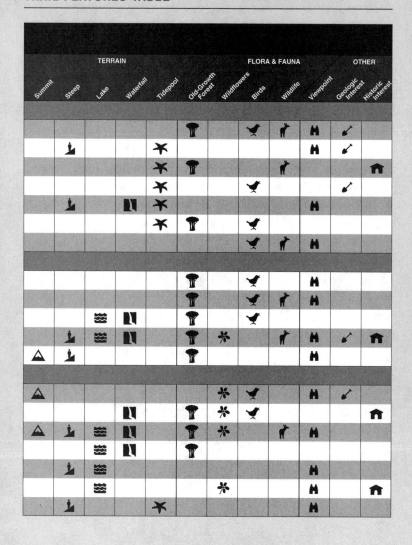

TRAIL FEATURES TABLE

Olympic National Park & Vicinity Trails

TRAIL NUMBER AND NAME	Page	Difficulty - 1 2 3 4 5+	Length in Miles	Type	Day Hiking	Backpacking	Mountain Biking	Horses	Dogs Allowed	Child-Friendly
4. North Central Region: Elwha and Hurricane Ridge Areas										
20 Griff Creek Trail to Rock Viewpoint	183	4	3.2	↗	🧍					
21 Goblins Gate–Geyser Valley Loop	187	3	5.9	↻	🧍	🎒		🐎		👫
22 Dodger Point	193	5	27.0	↗		🎒		🐎		
23 Lake Angeles and Klahhane Ridge Loop	200	4–5	7.4– 12.9	↺	🧍	🎒				
24 Cirque Rim Loop and Sunrise Ridge	207	1–2	1.1– 2.9	↻	🧍					👫
25 Hurricane Hill	213	2 and 4	3.2– 6.4	↗	🧍					👫
26 Elk Mountain	219	3	5.0	↗	🧍					👫
27 Grand Valley and Grand Pass Loop	224	5	13.9	↻	🧍	🎒				
5. Northeast Region: The Rain Shadow Area										
28 Dungeness Spit	243	3	10.8	↗	🧍					👫
29 Deer Ridge Trail	248	4	10.2	↗	🧍					
30 Baldy	254	5	8.2	↗	🧍					
31 Royal Basin	260	4–5	14.0– 15.8	↗	🧍	🎒				
32 Mount Townsend and Silver Creek Loop	266	5	7.6– 10.9	↺	🧍	🎒			🐕	
33 Mount Zion Ridge Viewpoint	274	3	4.6	↗	🧍		🚵	🐎	🐕	👫
34 Marmot Pass and Buckhorn Mountain	280	5	10.6– 12.4	↗	🧍	🎒			🐕	
35 Tunnel Creek Trail	286	4	9.2	↗	🧍				🐕	
6. Southeast Region: Duckabush and Skokomish Areas										
36 Ranger Hole and Murhut Falls	300	2	3.4	↗	🧍				🐕	👫
37 Lake of the Angels	305	5	7.4	↗	🧍	🎒				
38 Mount Ellinor	311	4	3.4	↗	🧍				🐕	
39 Staircase Rapids	317	1	1.8	↗	🧍					👫

TRAIL FEATURES TABLE

	TERRAIN						FLORA & FAUNA			OTHER		
Summit	Steep	Lake	Waterfall	Tidepool	Old-Growth Forest	Wildflowers	Birds	Wildlife	Viewpoint	Geologic Interest	Historic Interest
	●					●		●	●		
	●							●	●	●	●
●	●	●							●		●
	●	●			●	●			●	●	
●						●		●	●		
●	●					●		●	●		
	●					●			●		
●	●	●	●			●		●	●		
							●	●	●		●
●	●					●		●	●		
●	●					●			●		
	●	●	●		●	●			●		
●	●	●				●			●	●	
●	●					●			●		
●	●		●		●	●		●	●		
	●	●			●	●			●		●
	●		●							●	●
	●	●	●					●			●
●	●							●	●		
			●		●				●		

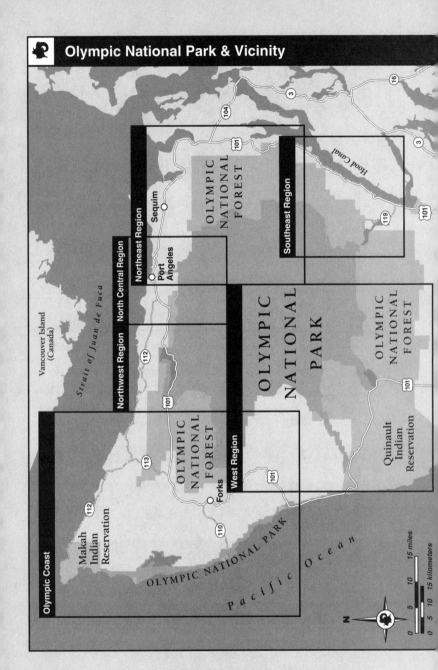

Olympic National Park & Vicinity

Contents

CHAPTER 1

Olympic Coast

CHAPTER 2

West Region: The Rain Forests

CHAPTER 3
Northwest Region:
Lake Crescent and Sol Duc Areas

CHAPTER 4
North Central Region:
Elwha and Hurricane Ridge Areas

CHAPTER 5
Northeast Region:
The Rain Shadow Area

CHAPTER 6
Southeast Region: Duckabush and Skokomish Areas

Using Top Trails™

Organization of Top Trails

Top Trails is designed to make identifying the perfect trail easy and to make every outing a success and a pleasure. With this book, you'll find that it's a snap to find the right trail, whether you're planning a major hike or just a sociable stroll with friends.

The Region

At the front of this book is the Olympic National Park & Vicinity Trail Features Table (pages iv–vii), which lists every trail covered in the guide, along with important attributes of each trip.

The following Olympic National Park & Vicinity Area Map (page viii) displays the entire area covered by this guide and provides a geographic overview. The map is clearly marked to show which area is covered by each

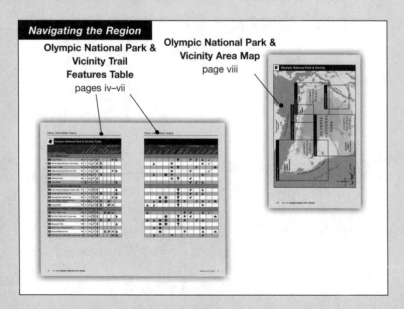

chapter. A quick reading of the regional map and the Trail Features Table
will give a good overview of the entire region covered by this guide.

The Areas

The region covered by this book is divided into six areas, with each chapter
corresponding to one area. Each area introduction contains information to
help you choose and enjoy a great trail every time out. To find the perfect
trip, use the table of contents or the regional map to identify your area of
interest, and then turn to the area chapter to find the following:

- An overview of the area, including maps and a general description of
  the terrain
- An area map with all featured trails clearly marked
- A trail features table providing trail-by-trail details
- Short trail summaries, written in an informative and accessible style

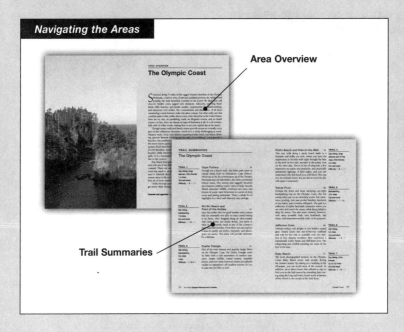

The Trails

The basic building block of the Top Trails guide is the trail entry. Each one
is arranged to make finding and following the trail as simple as possible,
with all pertinent information presented in an easy-to-follow format:

- A detailed trail map
- Trail descriptions covering difficulty, length, GPS coordinates, and other essential data
- A written trail text
- Trail milestones providing easy-to-follow, turn-by-turn trail directions

If the hike has substantial elevation gain and/or loss, the trail entry will also include an elevation profile.

In the margins of the trail entries, look for icons that point out notable features, such as viewpoints, wildflower displays, and wildlife-viewing locations at specific points along the trail.

Choosing a Trail

Top Trails provides several different ways of choosing a trail, using easy-to-read tables and maps.

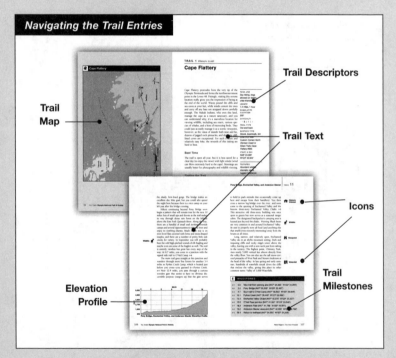

Navigating the Trail Entries

Trail Map

Trail Descriptors

Trail Text

Icons

Trail Milestones

Elevation Profile

Location

If you know in general where you want to go, Top Trails makes it easy to find the right trail in the right place. Each chapter begins with a large-scale map showing the starting point of every featured trail in that area.

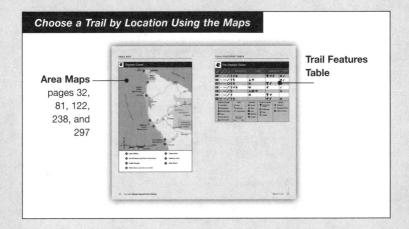

Choose a Trail by Location Using the Maps

Area Maps
pages 32,
81, 122,
238, and
297

Trail Features
Table

Features

This guide describes the top trails of Olympic National Park and vicinity, and each trail is chosen because it offers one or (usually) more features that make it especially appealing. Using the trail descriptors, summaries, and tables, you can quickly examine all the trails for the features they offer or seek a particular feature among the list of trails.

Season & Condition

Time of year and current conditions are often important factors in selecting the best trail. For example, an exposed hike in a timberline meadow may be filled with views and brightened by colorful wildflowers in midsummer, but it can be bitterly cold and dangerously windy in an autumn rain or snowstorm. Wherever relevant, Top Trails identifies the best and worst conditions for the trails you plan to hike.

Difficulty

Every trail has an overall difficulty rating on a scale of 1–5, which takes into consideration length, elevation change, exposure, and trail quality to create one (admittedly subjective) rating.

The ratings assume that you are an able-bodied adult in reasonably good shape, using the trail for hiking. The ratings also assume "good" weather conditions—mostly clear and dry (something that is far from a given on the Olympic Peninsula). Readers should make an honest assessment of their own abilities and adjust time estimates accordingly. Also, rain, snow, heat, wind, and poor visibility can all affect your pace on even the easiest of trails.

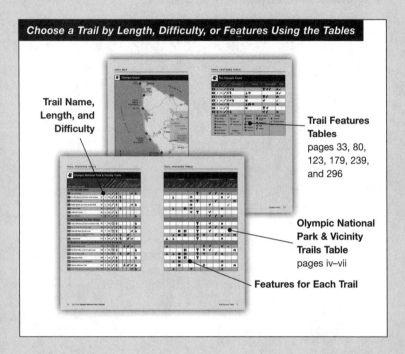

Choose a Trail by Length, Difficulty, or Features Using the Tables

Trail Name, Length, and Difficulty

Trail Features Tables
pages 33, 80, 123, 179, 239, and 296

Olympic National Park & Vicinity Trails Table
pages iv–vii

Features for Each Trail

Vertical Feet

Every trail description contains the approximate trail length and the overall elevation gain and loss over the course of the trail. It's important to use both figures when considering a hike. On average, plan nearly 1 hour of hiking for every 2 miles, and add as much as an hour for every 1,000 feet you climb.

The importance of elevation gains is often underestimated by hikers when gauging the difficulty of a trail. The Top Trails measurement accounts for *all* elevation change, not simply the difference between the highest and lowest points, so that rolling terrain with lots of up and down will be identifiable.

Top Trails Difficulty Ratings

1 A short trail, generally level, which can typically be completed in 1 hour or less.

2 A route of 1–3 miles, with some up and down, which can be completed in 1–2 hours.

3 A longer route, up to 5 or 6 miles, with some significant uphill and/or downhill sections.

4 A long or steep route, usually more than 5 miles, or with climbs of more than 1,000 vertical feet.

5 The most severe routes, both long and steep, more than 5 miles long and with climbs of 2,500 or more vertical feet. A few longer trails in this range may require backpacking.

The calculation of vertical feet in the Top Trails books is accomplished by a combination of trail measurement and computer-aided estimation. All of the routes in this book are either out-and-back hikes or loop trips that start and end at the same trailhead, so the total vertical elevation gain and loss are identical.

Finally, all trail entries with more than 1,000 feet of elevation gain include an elevation profile, an easy means for visualizing the topography of the route. These profiles graphically depict the elevation throughout the length of the trail.

Surface Type

Except for a handful of paved, gravel, or boardwalk routes, every inland trail in this book has a dirt surface. For beach routes, the surface typically consists of a short dirt or gravel access trail that leads to the shoreline, where you will walk on the sand and/or rocks. During this area's famously long (some would say unending) rainy season, or shortly after the snowmelt early in the summer, a dirt surface can turn into a muddy slog. Always choose the appropriate footwear to match the season and weather conditions.

Maps

Every trip in this book includes a map that is as up-to-date and accurate as possible. These maps use bold solid lines to indicate the featured trail and show all side trails and other relevant landmarks and geographic features.

Though this map will suffice for many easy and popular trails, you'll also need a good contour map for longer and more challenging trips. For most hikes, your best bet is to purchase one of the very hiker-friendly Custom Correct Maps that cover the relevant hiking region. The second best alternative is one (or more) of the Green Trails Maps. Unlike the Custom Correct Maps, however, where each map covers all the trails in a logical hiking area or zone, the Green Trails Maps are broken down by arbitrary latitude and longitude lines, which may cut right through your chosen hike. As a result, you sometimes have to purchase more than one Green Trails map to cover the full extent of your hike. Another alternative is to purchase the large Trails Illustrated map that covers all of Olympic National Park, though its scale means that this map lacks much of the detail of the Custom Correct or Green Trails Maps. The best available contour map for each hike is identified in the summary information at the start of the hike entry.

For hikes on Olympic National Forest land outside of the park, it will be helpful to purchase a copy of the *Olympic National Forest and National Park Map and Recreation Guide*. This will greatly assist in navigating the sometimes confusing system of roads on national forest land. Be aware, however, that the US Forest Service sometimes changes the road numbers, so the map may not always coincide with the signs on the ground.

Map Legend

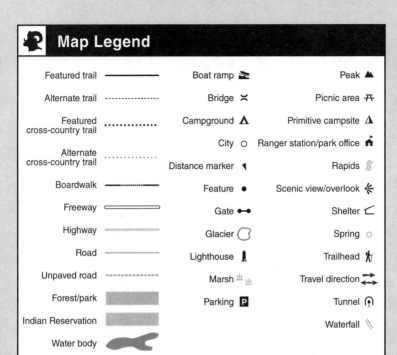

Featured trail	Boat ramp	Peak
Alternate trail	Bridge	Picnic area
Featured cross-country trail	Campground	Primitive campsite
Alternate cross-country trail	City	Ranger station/park office
Boardwalk	Distance marker	Rapids
Freeway	Feature	Scenic view/overlook
Highway	Gate	Shelter
Road	Glacier	Spring
Unpaved road	Lighthouse	Trailhead
Forest/park	Marsh	Travel direction
Indian Reservation	Parking	Tunnel
Water body		Waterfall
River/Stream		
Intermittent Stream		

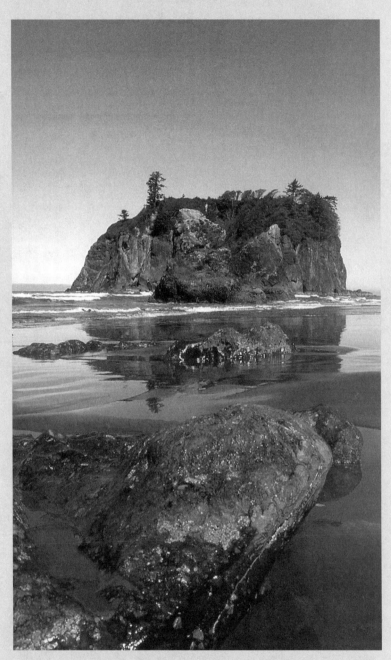

Abbey Island *at Ruby Beach (Trail 7)*

Introduction to Olympic National Park & Vicinity

L ocated in the far western part of Washington state, and forming the extreme western extension of the Lower 48, the Olympic Peninsula is a unique national treasure. As every visitor immediately notices, the land itself is rugged and scenic. It is also diverse, with everything from rocky shorelines and rain forests to alpine meadows and glacier-clad peaks. Some areas are even semideserts. Often these remarkably different landscapes are just a few miles apart. But the region is also unusual in its natural history. The peninsula is separated from the Cascade Mountains and other mountainous areas by the lowlands around Seattle and Puget Sound. Because this area has been isolated for at least 12,000 years, around the end of the Pleistocene era, numerous plants and animals on the peninsula have evolved separately from their distant relatives. This process has left the Olympic Peninsula with dozens of fascinating and endemic species that live nowhere else in the world. So, in effect, both time and Mother Nature have conspired to make the Olympic Peninsula a spectacular land apart.

In 1909 the federal government recognized this land's beauty and uniqueness when President Theodore Roosevelt set aside a portion of the peninsula's inland forests and mountains as the Mount Olympus National Monument. In part, this move was designed to protect the area's threatened elk herds, which were being hunted nearly to extinction. In fact, this preserve was almost named Elk National Park. The subspecies of elk that the great conservationist president was trying to protect was later named the Roosevelt elk, in his honor. In 1938 another Roosevelt (Franklin) signed into law the bill establishing Olympic National Park. A strip of magnificent coastline (the longest wild coastline in the Lower 48) was added to the park in 1953.

Geology

The rugged landscape of the Olympic Peninsula is not only spectacularly scenic, but it also has a fascinating geologic history that goes back millions of years. Although seemingly stable, that impressive landscape filling your camera viewfinder is actually undergoing constant change, and at such a relatively rapid pace that it is often possible for some fairly major changes to be noticeable in the lifetime of a single human being.

Even though they now tower nearly 8,000 feet above the nearby ocean, the Olympic Mountains were originally formed *under* the water. The rocks here are a complex mix of sedimentary rock (mostly sandstone and shale), which was laid down over millions of years as layers of sediment and mud under the ocean, and "pillow" basalts, which formed in a series of undersea volcanic eruptions. The rocks themselves are between 18 and 57 million years old—relatively young, in geologic terms. As the offshore oceanic plate that was carrying these rocks collided with the adjoining North American continental plate, fractures developed, and layers of this mix of rock pushed together and overrode each other. As the two great plates continued to grind toward one another, the rocks were tilted and forced upward. This, along with a general uplift of the area, is thought to have formed the mountains we see today. As the plates compressed against one another, they forced the new land to move in a generally northeasterly direction, forming a series of horseshoe-shaped bands of different rock types that wrap around the north, east, and south sides of the peninsula.

Erosion, by both streams and glaciers, carved the many deep canyons, broad valleys, and cirque basins of the range—a process that continues to this day. Today, however, the remaining glaciers are in rapid retreat, as temperatures have warmed and more of the area's prodigious precipitation falls as rain rather than snow. Comparison photographs show that all of the park's glaciers have shrunk in the last few decades, and some, such as the once large Lillian Glacier, have completely disappeared in the last 100 years.

Along the coast, erosion is even more evident. Waves are constantly crashing against the exposed headlands, carving into the base and slowly grinding these massive rocks into grains of sand. The countless offshore rocks that you pass while hiking the wilderness beaches represent former headlands of particularly hard rock that has, thus far, resisted its inevitable destruction. The placement of these rocks, sometimes miles offshore, is graphic evidence that the ocean is slowly winning this one-sided battle and the shoreline is in retreat. As with glaciers, comparison photos over just the last 100 years show dramatic and obvious changes to the shoreline as the rocks erode away and new headlands emerge.

Flora

The wide array of plants that now cover the rocks and soils of the Olympic Peninsula are at least as dramatic and beautiful as the geology underneath. The peninsula is home to more than 1,450 species of vascular plants, which is more than the entire British Isles, an area that is at roughly the same

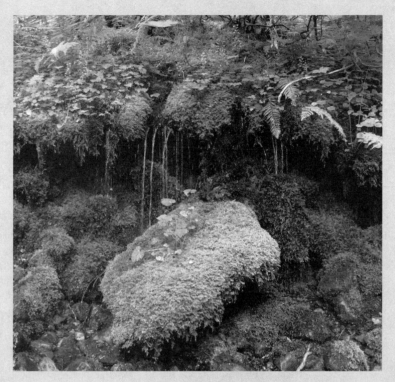

Dripping moss and ferns *along trail below Deer Lake on High Divide Loop (Trail 15)*

latitude and more than 30 times larger. And that impressive total excludes the hundreds of species of nonvascular plants, such as mosses, and the countless species of lichen and fungi, which are not true plants but are usually thought of that way.

But despite the great variety of species found here, what the typical hiker remembers most about his or her visit to the Olympic Peninsula, especially to the westside rain forests, is not the diversity but the overwhelming, almost unbelievable, *volume* of plant material found here. As you walk through these forests, you can't help but notice that everything, and I do mean *everything,* is green. The extremely dense overhead canopy is green. Every square inch of ground is carpeted with green. The tree trunks and tree limbs are draped with green. The downed logs have been taken over by green. Even the rocks are covered with green. Literally everything you can see, except, perhaps, the path you are walking on, is green. If there were a world capital for chlorophyll, then this would have to be it.

And this is not just the vague impression of a single, admittedly awed pedestrian: There are actual statistics to back this up. The temperate rain forests of the Olympic Peninsula support the greatest biomass of any eco-system on Earth. In simple terms, the total weight of living and once living material (primarily plants but also animals) is greater here than anywhere else on the planet. Even the famous Amazon rain forest in tropical South America has less than a third the total biomass in the same unit of area as the Olympic rain forests. To put it another way, what we basically have here is an incredibly dense, cool climate jungle.

Forests on the north and east sides of the range are much drier and less dense, but no less beautiful. And while the climate in high-elevation meadows and rock gardens is too harsh to support forests, they are home to a glorious wealth of wildflowers that enhance the beauty of any walk in this region on a summer day.

As with everything else on this diverse peninsula, the plant species you encounter depend largely on what part of the region you happen to be visiting.

In the low-elevation west-side rain forests, the dominant tree species are Sitka spruce and western hemlock. Interspersed with these massive trees are Douglas-fir and western red cedar and, near the river bottoms, deciduous trees, such as big-leaf maple and red alder. In places, the size of the grandest ancient conifers is awe inspiring, with many giants approaching 300 feet tall and with trunks that are as much as 60 feet in circumference. The most common shrub is salmonberry, which offers pretty lavender flowers in early spring and edible (but rather bland) berries in late summer. The abundant ground cover is a mix of, among others, oxalis, sword fern, lady fern, deer fern, and a host of mosses, lichens, and liverworts. Attached to the tree trunks and branches are numerous species of epiphytes, plants that grow on other plants. Included in this group are licorice fern, spike moss, lungwort, and numerous lichens that all add up to more displays of green than Crayola ever dreamed possible.

Douglas-fir dominates the mid-elevation forests on the west side of the peninsula, as well as the drier forests on the north and east sides of the range. Other common trees, depending on elevation, include Pacific madrone, Pacific silver fir, Alaska yellow cedar, lodgepole pine, and western hemlock. The most abundant shrubs in this environment are Oregon grape, several species of huckleberry, red elderberry, devil's club (especially in wet areas), and salal. Of special note in the drier eastern part of the range is the Pacific rhododendron, Washington's state flower. In June, the abundant pink blossoms of this tall shrub put on a magnificent show.

At the highest elevations, just below timberline, cold temperatures, heavy snowfall, and strong winds often stunt the forests. The tortured trees in this environment are usually mountain hemlock, Alaska yellow cedar, and subalpine fir.

In addition to the trees and shrubs, hundreds of other plant species fill the wide variety of ecological niches found on the Olympic Peninsula. The

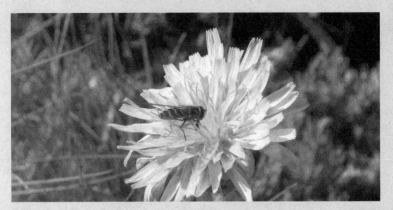

Bee *on flower blossom*

favorite group for most visitors is the wide assortment of colorful wildflowers that put on such a fine show April–mid-August, depending on the elevation.

A complete list of even the area's common wildflowers is beyond the scope of this book (not to mention the expertise of this author). In general, though there are some lovely wildflowers growing at low elevations, the best displays are found in the mid- and high-elevation meadows. Some of the most abundant varieties include:

BLUE AND PURPLE
broadleaf lupine, Olympic violet (endemic), larkspur, bluebells, aster, Flett's violet (endemic), Piper's bellflower (endemic), various penstemons

RED/PINK AND ORANGE
Indian paintbrush, pink mountain heath, shooting star, tiger lily, coralroot, smooth douglasia, spreading phlox (sometimes almost white), Lewis's monkeyflower, spirea, bleeding heart

WHITE
twinflower, avalanche lily, American bistort, bear grass, bunchberry, partridge-foot, spring beauty, goatsbeard, white mountain heather

YELLOW
yellow violet, alpine goldenrod, mountain arnica, Olympic Mountain groundsel (endemic), skunk cabbage (in low-elevation bogs), yellow monkeyflower, buttercup

Obviously with all of these different varieties, a good wildflower identification guide will come in handy.

Fauna

Olympic National Park is home to an assortment of wildlife habitats, probably more than any other unit in the national park system. No other preserve, after all, can boast of including within its borders everything from coastal beaches and tide pools to towering mountains draped with glaciers, from drenched temperate rain forests drowning in more than 14 *feet* of rain per year to semideserts eking out less than 20 inches of the wet stuff. And in each of these beautiful environments (as well as all the mixed bag of stuff in between), there is an equally wide assortment of animal life. When you throw in the fact that the Olympic Mountains' isolation has led to a number of animal species that live nowhere else in the world, you have a wildlife lover's paradise. In my more than 33,000 miles of hiking and backpacking through every corner of the American West, only Yellowstone National Park has provided more wildlife encounters than the Olympic Peninsula.

As with everything else in this diverse region, the types of animals you see depends on which environment you happen to be visiting.

On the coast, where wildlife is probably more easily observed than anywhere else, you will find a wide assortment of oceangoing mammals,

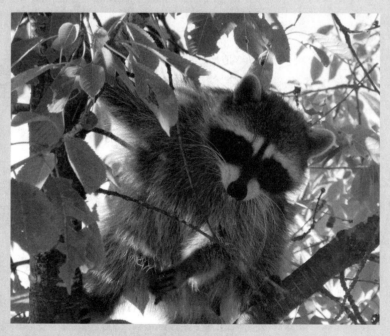

Raccoon (*a common thief along the Olympic Coast*)

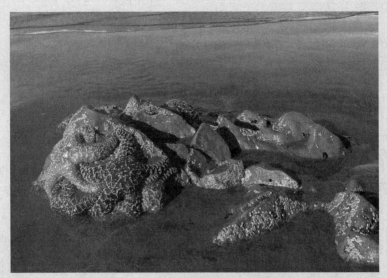

Sea stars *on beach rock in Jefferson Cove (Trail 6)*

including dolphins, various whales (gray, minke, killer, and others), harbor seals, sea lions, and otters (both river and sea). Of special note among the mammals of the forests and beaches *beside* the coastal zone is the ubiquitous raccoon. Although they are rarely seen on inland trails, near the coast this ever-curious and invariably hungry animal is extremely abundant. Their numbers and voracious appetites force backpackers to guard food *very* carefully.

Birds are also abundant and easily observed along the shoreline. It is not unusual to see as many as a dozen bald eagles a day while hiking the wilderness beaches. Other common coastal birds include black oyster catchers, sanderlings, rock sandpipers, three species of scoters (a kind of almost black, oceangoing duck), various gulls, three species of cormorants, rhinoceros auklets, pigeon guillemots, common murres, marbled murrelets, tufted puffins, ospreys, and common ravens.

The tidepools on the coast host a tremendous variety of colorful critters, and many people enjoy observing these animals. You can't miss the many sea stars (often called starfish), sea urchins, mussels, crabs, limpets, barnacles, small fish, and other beings that inhabit these resource-rich pools. Very fortunate individuals may even run across a more exotic animal, such as an octopus.

Mammals commonly encountered on inland trails range from the very large (Roosevelt elk) to the really tiny (shrews, mice, and chipmunks). Among the more common smaller mammals you are likely to see are the snowshoe hare, Douglas's squirrel, spotted skunk, and, if you are very

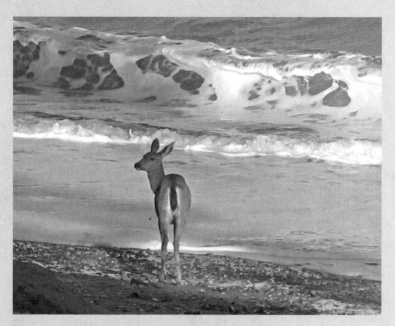

Deer on beach *at Dungeness Spit (Trail 28)*

lucky, mountain beaver (a pudgy and slow-moving fur bearer that is usually only active at night). The whistling and cute-as-a-button Olympic marmot is the best known of the endemic mammals here, and hikers who frequent the high-elevation trails often encounter these critters. Other endemic animals, such as the Olympic snow mole and Olympic chipmunk, are seldom seen by the casual observer. In 2008 fishers, a member of the weasel family, were reintroduced into Olympic National Park after being trapped to local extinction in the early part of the 20th century.

As for large mammals, both deer and elk are abundant, and you are very likely to see them. Deer are especially common in meadows early in the morning, while elk inhabit both the west-side rain forests and the high mountain meadows. Black bears are very common, especially in the park. In a few places and at certain times of the year, it is difficult to hike for more than a few hours *without* seeing one. On a hike in the early fall along the High Divide, for example, I encountered 14 black bears in one day! (Hence the park has strict rules requiring backpackers to secure their food from the bruins.) Although in other parts of the country black bears come in a range of colors, all of the bears in the Olympic Mountains are jet black. Scientists estimate that there are more mountain lions in Olympic than in any other national park, but these magnificent big cats are shy and rarely seen.

Of interest not by their presence but rather by their absence are a host of animals that are (or were) found in all other mountainous regions in the Pacific Northwest, but which never made it across the Puget Sound lowlands to colonize the Olympics. This list includes grizzly bears, bighorn sheep, red foxes, pikas, wolverines, lynx, white-tailed ptarmigans, and golden-mantled ground squirrels.

A final inland mammal that is worth special mention is the mountain goat. Although not native to the Olympic Mountains, these animals were introduced into the range in the 1920s before the park was established. The animals thrived, and their population exploded. Unfortunately, the Olympic ecosystem had not evolved to accommodate these hungry and invasive guests, and their sharp hooves and voracious appetites caused enormous damage to the fragile alpine plants. Getting rid of the invaders has proven to be extremely difficult and prohibitively expensive. Problems range from the inevitable budget concerns to loud cries by some to leave the creatures alone and just let nature take its course (conveniently ignoring the fact that nature has already been thrown *off* course by man). You may still see goats in the high country, and in a few places habituated animals are becoming a safety concern to hikers. Although intermittent efforts to remove the animals continue, in recent years the National Park Service thinks that, as one ranger told me, "Well, unfortunately, they're here now, and we just have to live with them."

Very few species of reptiles are found in the park, as these animals usually prefer drier climates. The only species of lizard known to occur here is the northern alligator lizard, and very few visitors ever see one. Snakes are a more common occurrence, with the rubber boa and two species of garter snake occasionally making appearances along the trails.

Unlike reptiles, the more water-loving amphibians are quite common. Several species of frogs, including the Pacific tree frog, red-legged frog, tailed frog, and Cascades frog, are found near freshwater throughout the peninsula. In drier areas, you may be fortunate enough to spot a western toad. Newts and salamanders are also abundant, with at least eight species found in the park. Perhaps the most interesting, if not the most common, is the Olympic torrent salamander, which is another endemic species found only on the Olympic Peninsula. This small (less than 5 inches long) salamander prefers cold mountain streams and can often be found living in the spray of waterfalls. Their coloration is medium to dark brown on the top and sides and bright yellow on the belly, often with some darker spots.

There are 37 species of native fish inhabiting the inland waters of the Olympic Peninsula, including the tiny Olympic mudminnow, yet another endemic species. For most visitors, the most impressive and exciting fish are the steelhead and five species of salmon that migrate up from the ocean into the peninsula's clear rivers and streams to spawn. There are numerous salmon runs at different times of the year, so you stand a reasonably good chance of seeing at least some fish moving upstream at almost any time during the hiking season. Black bears, river otters, bald eagles, and other animals rely on these fish as a vital source of protein, and the dead bodies of the fish after they spawn deposit important nutrients that help enrich the streams. The salmon runs on the Olympic Peninsula are some of the healthiest remaining for these troubled species, which I hope will soon get even healthier. The removal of the Glines Canyon Dam on the Elwha River, which since 1911 has blocked all salmon from reaching the upper river, will reopen 70 miles of long-lost spawning habitat for chinook and other salmon on one of the peninsula's largest rivers. In the planning stages for decades, the dam removal began in 2011 and is scheduled to be complete by September 2014. Once the dam is gone, it is hoped that the Elwha River's salmon, which once were known to be among the largest on Earth, with many fish exceeding 100 pounds, will eventually rebound from the current approximately 3,000 fish to something closer to the former historic totals of around 400,000.

Weather and When to Go

When giving speeches or presentations about the Olympic Peninsula, I often quip that other guidebook authors frequently say that the weather on the Olympic Peninsula is unpredictable. But that's not true. The weather on the Olympic Peninsula is very predictable. It's *bad*—downright miserable, in fact, a large part of the time. That comment fits the stereotype for this area and is always good for a laugh, but it's also not entirely true.

First of all, while not exactly arid, parts of the Olympic Peninsula are remarkably dry. The rainstorms in this part of the world come off the Pacific Ocean, usually in a path that leads the fronts from southwest to northeast. As a result, the northeast part of the peninsula sits in the rain shadow of all those peaks to the south and west, which conveniently soak up the vast majority of the moisture. Thus, while the west-side rain forests may receive more than 14 feet of rain per year, and Mount Olympus regularly gets as much as *200 feet* of snow, the valleys on the northeast side of the peninsula around the town of Sequim receive only about 17 inches of rain. It is not uncommon for hikers in this area to be bathed in sunshine while pedestrians just 40 miles to the southwest are drowning in heavy rainfall. The mountains above Sequim, in the northeast corner of the range, get more rain and snow than the valleys but still a lot less than peaks of the same elevation to the west.

Secondly, there is a seasonal element to the rain. Most of the precipitation (though not, unfortunately, *all* of it) falls from about mid-September to early June. Although that fills the majority of the calendar year, it still leaves a window of opportunity for relatively dry hiking mid-June–mid-September. It

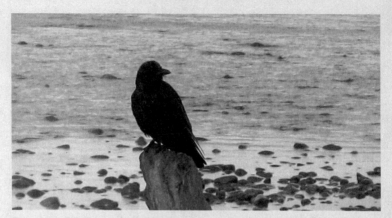

Raven *near Hoh River*

is not uncommon in July and August, for example, to get a solid week or two of dry and sunny weather, even on the soggy west side of the range.

Third, as with all rules, there are always exceptions. Sure, the average winter or spring day is rainy, but by no means does this apply to *every* day. In fact, every winter there are stretches of remarkably dry and sunny skies when hiking is a joy. And, on average, there are even more dry days in the spring and fall. About one year in three sees long periods of Indian summer in October, when the skies remain mostly clear and the temperatures cool. Of course this point about exceptions to the rule applies to summer as well, so even though summer is the driest part of the year, days (sometimes several in a row) of rain are not uncommon, and hikers need to be prepared.

Finally, a host of microclimates on the peninsula have a significant impact on the weather. Right along the beach, for example, typically gets significantly less rain (but more wind) than just a mile or two inland. Valleys and coastlines on the north side of the peninsula around Lake Crescent are often much drier than similar locations just a few miles to the west. Lastly, coastal fog and low clouds are common in the summer and early fall. The fog usually hugs the immediate coast, while the low clouds often push inland into the lower elevations of the river valleys and are sometimes thick enough to produce drizzle or even light rain. These clouds frequently burn off by late in the day, and if you climb above 3,000 feet or so, you will typically find yourself above the clouds and amid brilliant sunshine.

A final positive aspect of the local weather is that the peninsula's closeness to the moderating influence of the Pacific Ocean keeps temperatures very mild. It is extremely rare, for example, for temperatures to reach above 85°F anywhere on the peninsula even for a day or two. Highs in the comfortable mid-60s to mid-70s are the norm, even in midsummer.

And even in the worst winters, temperatures at lower elevations are rarely much below freezing, and snow is uncommon (and usually only transitory) below 1,000 feet.

All of this means that, despite the famously rainy climate, the Olympic Peninsula offers outstanding hiking at any time of the year. Locals recognize, for example, that those occasional dry winter days are excellent times to hit the trails and enjoy some uncrowded hiking. The beach routes are always open, and low-elevation rain forest trails are also generally available for hiking in the winter, except during those very rare low-elevation snow and ice events that temporarily close roads and trails. Another important point is that even if it is raining, you should not be discouraged and stay off the trails. With good raingear and the right attitude, there are dozens of outstanding hikes on the peninsula that are just as much fun (sometimes even *more* fun) in wet and cloudy weather as they are under sunny skies. A walk through dense forest to a waterfall, for example, does not require sunshine to be enjoyed. The forest will protect you from the worst of the weather, and amid the trees you won't be missing any views. Similarly, not only does hiking in a rain forest when it is raining have a certain appropriate symmetry to it, but the rain also makes the greens of the mosses and other plants more vibrant and beautiful.

That being said, rest assured that I am *not* one of those hiking masochists who deliberately hits the trails even in the worst weather to fully experience nature (or some such similar nonsense). Frankly, trudging along in a driving rainstorm with 50-mile-per-hour winds and temperatures in the high 30s is not my idea of fun. Thus, when I say that hiking in the rain on the Olympic Peninsula can be enjoyable, I mean when it is a fairly light rain with moderate temperatures and winds—the norm around here. Now *that* can be fun. Take this non-masochist's word for it.

Shoulder season hiking, in the spring and fall, is equally rewarding. There are few crowds, permits for the backcountry are usually easy to obtain, and often the wildlife is easier to see. At low elevations, the forest wildflowers start blooming in early April, and there are nice fall colors in both the lowland valleys (maples and cottonwoods) and the subalpine meadows (huckleberries) in October. Keep in mind, however, that shoulder season hikers should be prepared for extended periods of wet weather.

Summer is prime season for hiking at any elevation on the peninsula, with the best chance for good weather. The snows at the highest elevations typically melt by mid- to late July, and this is soon followed by the parade of colorful alpine and subalpine wildflowers. Of course, many other people feel the same way about summer, which is why the majority of Olympic National Park's 3 million annual visitors arrive June–early September. As a result, you can expect plenty of company, especially on popular trails. In addition, obtaining a backcountry permit for your preferred location may be difficult, though there are excellent alternatives if your first choice is unavailable.

Below, the table compares the average temperature and precipitation of Forks and Sequim for each month. The city of Forks in the rain forest section of the peninsula gets an annual average of 121.73 inches of precipitation, while Sequim in the northeast rain shadow area gets an average of just 16.06 inches. The temperature differences between the two places, however, are minimal, with both having quite mild temperatures year-round that differ on average only by a degree or two every month. But in December, January, and February, Forks averages more rain in any one of these months than Sequim gets all year! As the crow flies, the two cities are only a little more than 50 miles apart.

SEQUIM						
month	JAN	FEB	MAR	APR	MAY	JUNE
Hi Temp	45°F	48°F	52°F	56°F	61°F	65°F
Precipitation	1.89"	1.46"	1.22"	0.98"	1.18"	1.02"
month	JULY	AUG	SEPT	OCT	NOV	DEC
Hi Temp	69°F	69°F	65°F	58°F	50°F	46°F
Precipitation	0.67"	0.75"	0.83"	1.26"	2.56"	2.24"
FORKS						
month	JAN	FEB	MAR	APR	MAY	JUNE
Hi Temp	44°F	49°F	52°F	57°F	62°F	66°F
Precipitation	16.65"	15.47"	13.5"	8.98"	6.14"	3.82"
month	JULY	AUG	SEPT	OCT	NOV	DEC
Hi Temp	70°F	72°F	69°F	59°F	49°F	44°F
Precipitation	2.8"	2.76"	4.37"	11.06"	17.72"	18.46"

Trail Selection

Although this book includes a wide selection of the trails in Olympic National Park and vicinity, this is not a comprehensive listing of all the available hiking opportunities. Only the premier nature trails, day hikes, and a few longer overnight trips are included, based primarily on excellent scenery and diversity of experience for the hiker. Some of the selected trails are very popular, while others are rarely used. All of the trips are attractive and just plain fun, but for a subjective listing of what I believe to be the best of the best, see Appendix 1.

Trail Safety

The most common and serious danger to hikers on the Olympic Peninsula is hypothermia, the dangerous (potentially even deadly) loss of core body temperature. Given the local climate, you should be prepared for cold rain or, at higher elevations, snow at any time of year. The best plan for all but short walks on nice summer days is to be prepared with good raingear and several layers of warm clothing. Also, stay out of the wind, watch members of your party for symptoms of hypothermia (shivering, slurred speech, stumbling, and lack of manual dexterity), and always remain well hydrated. Treat mildly hypothermic persons by moving them to a sheltered area, getting them into dry clothing, and feeding them high-energy snacks and warm drinks. In more severe cases, skin-to-skin contact in a warm sleeping bag is the best plan. Remember that it does not have to be freezing for hypothermia to set in. In fact, most cases of hypothermia occur when temperatures are between 35° and 55°.

Winter storms are fierce in this area, so you can expect plenty of downed trees and washouts along trails and roads early in the hiking season. The park and surrounding forest do an admirable job of trying to keep on top of this situation, but it's a huge job, so plan to encounter some obstacles before the maintenance is complete. Always call ahead (or at least check the park's or national forest's website) about the latest road and trail closures. Nearly every winter, some roads are washed out and closed for at least a few days or weeks. A couple of roads have remained closed for years.

Brush grows ridiculously fast in this wet environment, so it frequently encroaches on the trails, especially routes that receive less use and maintenance. The plants themselves are generally harmless (there are very few sharp thorns like there are in desert country, there's not much in the way of poison oak, and only a few places have stinging nettles), but fighting through often-wet brush is tiring and can get you soaked, unless you are wearing raingear.

Coastal routes are associated with a unique set of hazards. Much of the hiking here is not on gentle sandy beaches but over rocks and boulders that are often unstable and/or covered with slippery seaweed. In addition, winter storms often scour away the sand that does exist, leaving behind rugged boulder fields and jagged-edged tide pools. All of this makes footing treacherous, and turned ankles are a real danger. Tides are another problem because they often block access around headlands, forcing hikers to either wait, possibly for hours, or to scramble over headlands using (when available) steep rope "ladders" that allow difficult overland passage. Finally, large "sneaker" waves occasionally sweep the beaches, washing away unwary hikers and/or moving huge drift logs that smash everything in sight. Always keep a close eye on the ocean and be extremely careful about your footing to ensure a safe hike.

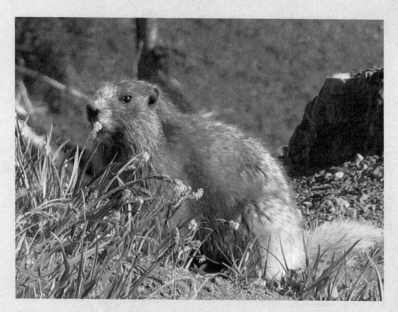

Olympic marmot

An often-overlooked hazard (well, really more of an annoyance) is spiderwebs. Several species of nonpoisonous arachnids use the narrow forest openings created by trails to hang their webs between the overhanging limbs and brush on either side. As a result, the first hiker on a trail in the morning will encounter dozens of webs smacking him or her across the face and body. Waving a walking stick in front of you helps, or you can employ my favorite strategy: following close behind an unknowing (and taller) hiking partner.

Mosquitoes and flies are an occasional nuisance, especially near smaller lakes, marshes, or any relatively wet area during the height of the bug season in early to midsummer. At lower elevations, you can expect mosquitoes to be common May–July, while the little vampires peak at upper elevations as the snow melts in July. By late summer and fall, most of the bugs are gone and the hiking is a joy.

An unusual risk on the trails in mid- to high-elevation meadows comes from marmots. These common animals usually place their burrow entrances in bare and open parts of meadows, so when the marmots emerge from underground, they can immediately spot any potential predators. As a result, the marmots often use the convenient openings of trails for their burrows. It is extremely easy for unwary hikers to step in one of these burrows and turn an ankle. When hiking through meadows, be sure to watch your step carefully to avoid this problem.

Thunderstorms are rare on the Olympic Peninsula, but they occasionally occur, especially in midsummer. If a thunderstorm is approaching, and especially if you see lightning anywhere in the area, head back to your car or into a densely forested area as quickly as possible.

Very few wild animals pose a potential danger to humans within the area covered by this book. Although hundreds of mountain lions prowl the forests and ridges here, they are almost never seen and attacks are virtually unknown. If you see a mountain lion, keep your children and pets nearby and try to intimidate the animal by standing tall and looking as big as possible. Mountain goats have become a problem in a few places, where they are habituated to humans and may approach very closely to hikers. This is a potentially dangerous situation, so hikers are reminded to stay at least 100 feet away from the animals and, if they approach you, to frighten them away by yelling, waving your arms, or throwing rocks. Finally, black bears are common and hikers see them fairly often. If you give the bears, especially a sow with cubs, a wide berth, the animals will generally ignore you. They can become a problem, however, especially near popular camping areas where the bears sometimes try to steal food. In several areas (Royal Basin, High Divide, the Sol Duc watershed, and Grand Valley), backpackers are required to store their food and garbage in bear canisters. Elsewhere, backpackers must either use a bear canister or, when trees are available, hang their food from a narrow tree limb at least 12 feet off the ground and 10 feet from the tree trunk. Car campers should keep all food in their vehicles.

Backpackers on coastal hikes face an even more common threat to their food supplies: raccoons. These abundant thieving rascals happily snatch up anything edible or otherwise interesting that is temporarily left unguarded or unsecured. To combat this menace, the National Park Service requires that coastal backpackers keep all food and other odorous items in hard-sided containers (a bear canister works) that are inaccessible to the raccoons. If you don't already have one, appropriate containers are available for loan/rent at ranger stations when you pick up your permit.

Key Features

Top Trails books contain extensive information about features for each trail, such as rain forests, tidepools, waterfalls, wildflowers, wildlife-viewing opportunities, places of historical interest, great viewpoints, and more. The Olympic Peninsula is blessed with such an incredible diversity of terrain, flora, and fauna that no matter what your interests, you are sure to find a trail to match them. Hikes in this book range from rugged seashore to stark ridges well above timberline and from drippy rain forests to amazingly dry meadows and open forests. If you are looking for a deep woods experience surrounded by a symphony of green or a view-packed walk on a high mountain, there is a great hike (in fact, *lots* of great hikes) here for you.

A wide assortment of campgrounds, historic lodges, and motels in town make for perfect base camps for days of great hiking. Countless backpacking options allow hikers to go farther, see more, and spend a memorable night or two under the stars. You can fish for salmon, poke around in tidepools, photograph acres of mountain wildflowers, visit a towering waterfall, watch a herd of elk, and enjoy a spectacular sunset all in the same day (no kidding—I've done it many times), or spend several glorious uninterrupted days really getting to know a single incredible ecosystem. Just find the feature, or the entire range of features, that most interests you and enjoy.

Multiple Uses

All the trails in this book were originally designed and built for hiking and remain excellent for that purpose. Many of the trails are equally good for jogging, though some are less suited for that purpose, either due to the rugged and rocky terrain or because they are very popular trails where jogging is difficult and may disturb other users.

In Olympic National Park, bicycles are allowed only on paved roads and are strictly prohibited on all trails except the Spruce Railroad Trail (Trail 18) on the north side of Lake Crescent. Similarly, bicycles are not allowed on national forest trails that travel through designated wilderness areas.

Hikers who like to take along their dogs have relatively limited options on the Olympic Peninsula. Pets are prohibited on all trails in the national park (except, again, the Spruce Railroad Trail) but are allowed on almost all trails in the surrounding national forests. Unfortunately, some US Forest Service trails are too rugged to recommend for dogs. Pets are also prohibited on all beach routes in the park, except for the lower end of Rialto Beach south of Ellen Creek (Trail 4) and the Kalaloch beaches south of Hoh River.

Finally, horses are allowed on nearly all trails on national forest land but only on a few select routes within Olympic National Park.

Fees & Permits

Olympic National Park charges all visitors an entrance fee. As of 2014, the fee was $15 per car and $5 for pedestrians, bicyclists, or motorcyclists (children age 15 and younger are admitted free). The pass is valid for entry into the park for seven consecutive days. American citizens and permanent residents 62 years or older can buy an Interagency Senior Pass for a *one-time* charge of just $10. This allows for lifetime entry to all national parks and other federal lands regardless of the agency in charge. (This has to be one of the best all-time

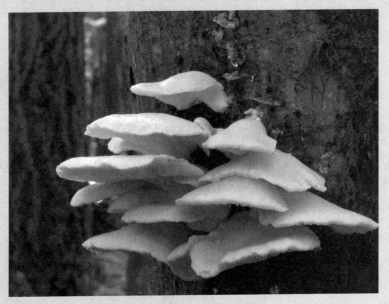

Mushrooms *on tree along Striped Peak Trail (Trail 19)*

deals since somebody offered Albert Einstein a penny for his thoughts.) Non-seniors can buy an annual Interagency Federal Recreational Lands Pass for $80 (as of 2014). This allows you entry for one year into not only all national parks and monuments but also all national wildlife refuges, Bureau of Land Management lands, US Forest Service lands, U.S. Fish and Wildlife Service lands, and Bureau of Reclamation lands. Conveniently, this pass works at trailheads in the Olympic National Forest that charge a parking fee. Without a Federal Recreational Lands Pass, you must have a Northwest Forest Pass to park at the more popular and developed US Forest Service trailheads. As of 2014, these passes—which you may obtain at all US Forest Service ranger stations, all Olympic National Forest offices, and some local sporting goods stores—cost $5 for a daily pass and $30 for an annual pass.

Not covered by any of the above are extra charges for special services or facilities, such as overnight fees to stay at car campgrounds. All of the dozens of developed National Park Service, US Forest Service, and county park car campgrounds in this area charge a fee, with the amount varying with the level of services provided. On US Forest Service land (but *not* in Olympic National Park), informal dispersed camping is allowed in most undeveloped areas and no fee is charged.

If you are hiking on Makah Indian Reservation lands (Trails 1 and 2 in this book), you must purchase a recreational use permit from the tribe. These are available from Washburn's General Store, the Makah Museum, and the Makah Tribal Center in Neah Bay. As of 2014, the charge was a very reasonable $10 for a pass that was good for the entire calendar year. Part of Trail 7 goes through the Hoh Indian Reservation, but the tribe allows hikers to have access to the beach without a permit.

No additional permit is required for day hiking anywhere on the peninsula, but backpackers staying overnight in Olympic National Park must have a backcountry use permit. As of 2014, these permits cost $5 for groups up to 12 persons with an additional charge of $2 per person per night. There is no additional per-night charge for children age 15 and younger. Frequent wilderness users may save money by purchasing an annual backcountry pass for $30.

When there is no limit on the number of people allowed to camp in an area of Olympic National Park, all you have to do is pick up a permit at a nearby ranger station or from the Wilderness Information Center in Port Angeles on the day of your trip and pay the fee.

A few of the more popular places in the park have limited entry backcountry permits that are required between May 1 and September 30. Somewhat confusingly, the rules differ for each area. Some places in the park (for example, Grand Valley and High Divide) have about half of the available permits available for reservations, with the rest set aside on a first-come, first-serve basis, and they are obtainable at the nearest Wilderness Information Center or ranger station. For other areas (for example, Royal Basin and the Ozette Triangle), permits are *only* given to people who make advanced reservations. To apply for a reservation, visit the park's website (**nps.gov/olym**), download a Wilderness Camping Permit Reservation Request form, fill out your information and planned itinerary, include your payment, and then send it by snail mail (see Appendix 2) or fax (360-565-3108) to the Wilderness Information Center. Reservation requests are accepted starting on March 15 of each calendar year.

The permitting requirements (if any) for each area in this book are outlined in the summary information for the individual trip.

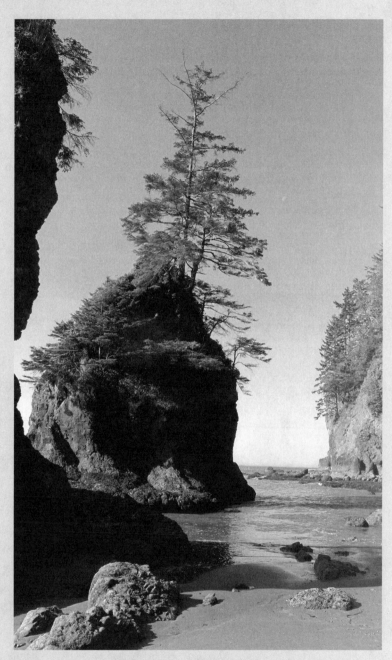

Rock pinnacle *in cove south of Taylor Point (Trail 5)*

On the Trail

E very outing should begin with proper preparation. Even the easiest trail can have surprises. People seldom think about getting lost or injured, but unexpected things can and do happen. Simple precautions can make the difference between a good story and a potentially dangerous situation.

Use the Top Trails ratings and descriptions to determine if a particular trail is a good match with your fitness and energy level, given current conditions and the time of year.

Have a Plan

Choose wisely The first step to enjoying any trail is to match the trail to your abilities. It's no use overestimating your experience or fitness. Know your abilities and accept your limitations, and then use the Top Trails Difficulty Rating that accompanies each trail to find a good fit.

Leave word about your plans The most basic precaution is leaving word of your intentions with friends or family. Many people will hike the backcountry their entire lives without ever relying on this safety net, but establishing this simple habit is good (and free) insurance.

It's best to leave specific information, including location, trail name, and intended time of travel, with a responsible person. However, if this is not possible or if plans change at the last minute, you should still try to leave word. If there is a wilderness registration process available, make use of it. If there is a ranger station, trail register, or visitor center, check in.

Review the route Before embarking on any hike, read the entire description and study the map. It isn't necessary to memorize every detail, but it is worthwhile to have a clear mental picture of the trail and the general area.

If the trail or terrain is long or complex, augment the trail guide with a topographic map. Maps and current weather and trail information are often available from local ranger and park stations, and these resources should be utilized (see Appendix 2).

Prepare and Plan

- Know your abilities and limitations.
- Leave word about your plans.
- Know the area and the route.

Carry the Essentials

Proper preparation for any type of trail use includes gathering certain essential items to carry. Trip checklists will vary tremendously by trail and conditions.

Clothing When the weather is good, light, comfortable clothing is the obvious choice. It's easy to believe that very little spare clothing is needed, but a prepared hiker has something tucked away for any emergency, from a surprise shower to an unexpected overnight in a more remote area.

Clothing includes proper footwear. As a trail becomes more demanding, you will need footwear that performs. Running shoes are fine for many shorter and easy trails when the sun is shining. If you will be carrying substantial weight or encountering either sustained rugged terrain or muddy trails from rain or snow, step up to hiking boots.

In hot, sunny weather, especially on an exposed trail, proper clothing includes a hat, sunglasses, long-sleeved shirt, and sunscreen. In cooler weather, particularly when it's wet (and those two frequently go together on the Olympic Peninsula), carry waterproof outer garments and quick-drying undergarments (avoid cotton). As a general rule, whatever the conditions, bring layers that can be combined or removed to provide comfort and protection from the elements in a wide variety of conditions.

Water Even though water is generally an abundant resource on the Olympic Peninsula, you should never set out on a trail without some drinking water. At all times, particularly in warm weather, adequate water is of key importance. Experts recommend at least 2 quarts of water per full day on the trail, and when hiking in heat, a gallon or more may be appropriate. At the extreme, dehydration can be life threatening. More commonly, inadequate water brings fatigue and muscle aches.

For most outings, unless the day is very hot or the trail very long, you should carry sufficient water for the entire trip. Drinking directly from natural water sources is *not* recommended because these are often contaminated with bacteria, viruses, and other nasty microscopic critters that can make your life absolutely *miserable* (take this giardia victim's word for it).

Trail Essentials

- Dress to keep cool, but be ready for cold.
- Bring plenty of water and adequate food.

Water treatment If you are backpacking or on an extremely long day hike in hot weather, it will be necessary to make use of trailside water. All such water should be treated before use. There are four methods for treating water: boiling, chemical treatment, ultraviolet light treatment, and filtering. Boiling is very effective but often impractical because it requires a heat source, a pot, and time. Chemical treatments, available at most outdoor stores, handle some problems, including the troublesome giardia parasite, but will not combat cryptosporidium or many man-made chemical pollutants. Most hikers prefer ultraviolet light treatment and filtration. Both methods effectively kill or remove giardia and other microscopic nasties and leave no unpleasant aftertaste.

Food While not as critical as water, food is energy and its importance should not be underestimated. Avoid foods that are hard to digest, such as candy bars and potato chips. Carry high energy, fast-digesting foods: nutrition bars, dehydrated fruit, jerky, and/or trail mix. Always bring a little extra food—it's good protection against an outing that turns unexpectedly long, perhaps due to weather or losing your way.

Useful but Less than Essential Items

Navigation devices (and the know-how to use them) Many trails don't require much navigation, meaning a map and compass or GPS device aren't always as essential as water or food, but it's a close call. If the trail is remote or infrequently visited, or if you plan to do any off-trail travel, a contour map and compass or GPS device should be considered necessities. And remember that a GPS is not a substitute for a map. After all, knowing your exact longitude and latitude is not much help without a good map.

In addition, it is worth noting that the incredibly dense forests, especially on the west side of the Olympic Peninsula, pose a unique problem for hikers using a GPS. There is probably nowhere else on the planet with a thicker overhead forest canopy than this environment, so it can be difficult for your GPS to lock onto a satellite (much less two or three) and obtain a reading. Once you climb above the trees, it's not a problem, but in the forests, using a GPS for navigation ranges from difficult to impossible.

Cell phone Although most parts of the country have some level of cellular coverage, in many of the remote areas around the Olympic Peninsula, it will be impossible to obtain a signal. Do not depend on your cell phone to get you out of a jam. In addition, even if you can get service, be sure that the occasion warrants a phone call. A blister doesn't justify a call to search and rescue.

Gear Depending on the remoteness and rigor of the trail, there are many additional useful items to consider: pocketknife, flashlight, fire source (waterproof matches, light, or flint), a warm knit cap, an emergency signaling whistle, and a first-aid kit.

Every member of your party should carry the appropriate essential items described above because groups often split up or get separated along the trail. Solo hikers should be even more disciplined about preparation and carry more gear. Traveling solo is inherently more risky. This isn't meant to discourage all solo travel, especially for experienced hikers, but simply to emphasize the need for extra preparation.

Trail Etiquette

The overriding rule on the trail is "Leave No Trace." Interest in visiting natural areas continues to increase in North America, even as the quantity of unspoiled natural areas continues to shrink. These pressures make it ever more critical that we leave no trace of our visits.

Never litter If you carried it in, it's easy enough to carry it out. Leave the trail in the same (preferably even better) condition that you find it. Try picking up any litter you encounter and packing it out—it's a great feeling! Just one piece of garbage and you've made a difference.

Camp responsibly Backpackers need to be especially careful to be gentle on the land. Always put up your tent in a designated site or a place that is either compacted from years of previous use or can easily take the impact without being damaged—sand, rocks, or a densely wooded area is best. *Never* camp on fragile meadow vegetation or immediately beside a lake or stream. If you

---

 Trail Etiquette

- Leave no trace. Never litter.
- Stay on the trail. Never cut switchbacks.
- Share the trail. Use courtesy and common sense.
- Leave it there.
- Don't disturb wildlife.

---

see a campsite "growing" in an inappropriate location, be proactive: Place a few limbs or rocks over the area to discourage further use, scatter "horse apples," and remove any fire-scarred rocks. In designated wilderness areas, regulations generally require that you camp at least 100 feet from water.

Do not build campfires. Although fires were once a staple of camping and backpacking, today few areas can sustain the negative impact of fires. For cooking, use a lightweight stove (they are more reliable, easier to use, and cleaner than fires), and for warmth, try wearing a sweater or going for an evening stroll. In Olympic National Park and most US Forest Service wilderness areas, fires are prohibited above 3,500 feet.

Finally, backpackers should leave both of the following at home: soap (even biodegradable soap pollutes; just throw water over yourself to remove the daily dirt) and any outdated attitudes you may have about going out to conquer the wilderness.

Stay on the trail The established trails have been created for many purposes: to protect the surrounding natural areas, to avoid dangers, and to provide the best route. Leaving the trail can cause damage that takes years to undo. Never cut switchbacks. Shortcutting rarely saves energy or time, and it takes a terrible toll on the land, trampling plant life and hastening erosion. Moreover, safety and consideration intersect on the trail. It's hard to get truly lost if you stay on the trail.

Share the trail The best trails often attract many visitors, and you should be prepared to share the trail. Do your part to minimize impact. Commonly accepted trail etiquette dictates that **bike riders yield to both hikers and equestrians, hikers yield to horseback riders, downhill hikers yield to uphill hikers, and everyone stays to the right.** Not everyone knows these rules of the road, however, so let common sense and good humor be your guide.

Leave it there Destruction or removal of plants and animals, or historical, prehistoric, or geological items, is certainly unethical and almost always illegal. Hikers are allowed to collect and eat wild berries, but only in small quantities and for personal consumption.

Getting lost To avoid getting lost while hiking, the best plan is to always try to stay on the trail. Sometimes confusing game trails or faint routes may cause you to lose the correct route. Stop and take stock of the situation. In many cases, a few minutes of calm reflection will yield a solution and a way to relocate the proper route. Consider all the clues available, and use the sun to identify directions if you don't have a compass. If you determine that you are indeed lost, it is usually best to stay put. You are more likely to encounter other people if you stay in one place.

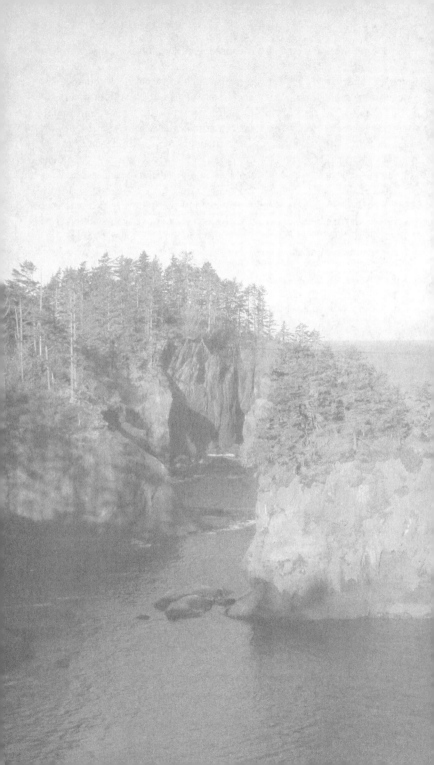

Olympic Coast

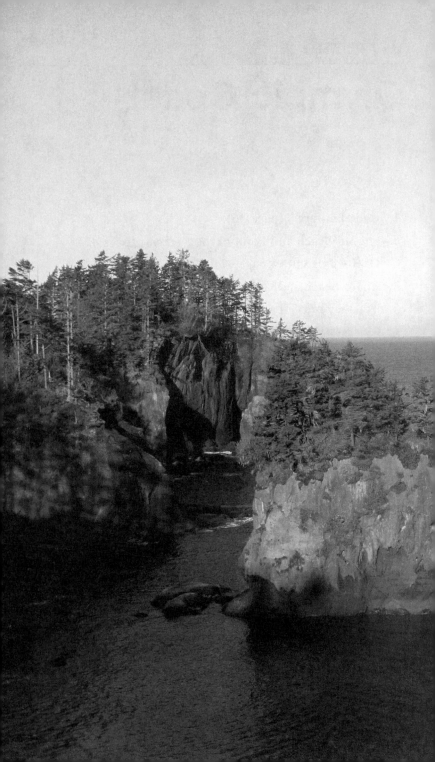

The Olympic Coast

Stretched along 73 miles of the rugged western shoreline of the Olympic Peninsula, a narrow strip of national parkland protects the wildest (and possibly the most beautiful) coastline in the Lower 48. Here, you will discover hidden coves, jagged rock pinnacles, tidepools, towering headlands, cliffs, beaches, spectacular sunsets, opportunities for beachcombing, and numerous rock arches. The concentration and abundance of all these outstanding coastal features make this place unique, but what really sets this coastline apart is that, unlike almost every other shoreline in the United States, there are no cars, no paralleling roads, no lifeguard towers, and no beach resorts—in fact, there are almost no signs of humanity at all. It is all wonderfully wild. In other words, visiting here is not your typical day at the beach.

Though scenic trails and beach routes provide access to virtually every part of this wilderness shoreline, much of it is fairly challenging to reach. Slippery rocks, steep rope ladders requiring tricky hand-over-hand climbing (picture Batman climbing up the side of a building), wave-pounded beaches, tide problems, and the inevitable weather issues all make hiking the more remote parts of this wilderness shoreline a challenge. Still, backpackers flock here for the experience of a lifetime—walking mile after mile of wild shoreline, scrambling over headlands, and camping on uncrowded beaches while listening to the lapping of waves and the squawking of gulls. It is a backpacking experience that is unknown almost anywhere else in the country.

Day hikers find great sport here as well, and they usually don't have to deal with any of the difficult access issues with which overnight hikers must contend. There are numerous excellent day hikes accessed by dead-end roads that reach to, or nearly to, the ocean. The longest stretch of unbroken sand is Kalaloch Beach in the south, with easy access off US 101. More remote areas to the north offer much more dramatic and varied scenery, so they are of more interest to the average hiker.

Unlike the high country, the beaches can be hiked all year, though it can get pretty bleak during winter storms. Locals usually prefer the off-season

Overleaf and opposite: *Cove on west side of Cape Flattery (Trail 1)*

because they don't have to contend with either the tourists or the fog, both of which tend to crowd the immediate coastline for much of the summer. Probably the best compromise is to visit during the shoulder seasons of spring and fall, when crowds are few, the wildlife is easy to see, the fog is not a problem, and the coastal scenery is sublime. With that in mind, a joke in these parts holds that native Northwesterners are often mystified to learn that people in other parts of the world actually take *off* layers of clothing when they visit the beach. Unless you're into tanning your goose bumps, nobody does that here. Come prepared with clothing that will keep you comfortable in cool and windy weather, even in midsummer when it (probably) isn't raining.

Remember to check the tide tables before you set out. Low tide may be required to safely round some headlands. In addition, a lower tide makes for easier hiking on hard-packed wet sand—and for more enjoyment as you explore tidepools. Tide charts are available at local ranger stations and sporting goods stores, or they can be downloaded from the Internet. One of the best sources is the website for the National Oceanic and Atmospheric Administration at **www.tidesandcurrents.noaa.gov.**

Finally, be aware that though exploring tidepools is rewarding and enormously fun, please leave the colorful but fragile creatures who live there undisturbed.

Governing Agencies

Most of the Olympic Coast is administered by Olympic National Park, but the far northern portion (Trail 1 and part of Trail 2) is on the Makah Indian Reservation, and part of the shoreline north of Ruby Beach (Trail 7) is on the Hoh Indian Reservation.

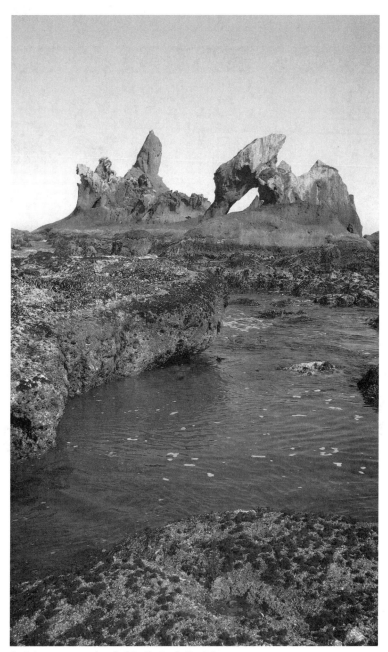

Arch in cove *at north end of Shi Shi Beach (Trail 2)*

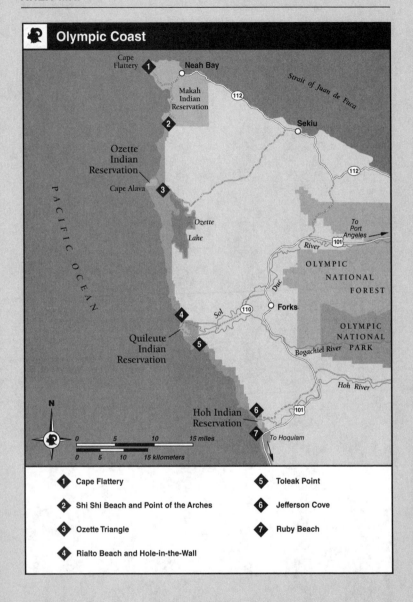

Olympic Coast

Cape
Flattery **1** **Neah Bay**

Strait of Juan de Fuca

Makah
Indian
Reservation

112

2

Sekiu

Ozette
Indian
Reservation

Cape Alava **3**

PACIFIC OCEAN

*Ozette
Lake*

To
Port
Angeles

Duc River 101

OLYMPIC

NATIONAL

FOREST

4 *Sol* 110 **Forks**

OLYMPIC
NATIONAL
PARK

Quileute
Indian
Reservation

5

Bogachiel River

Hoh River

N

0   5   10   15 miles

0   5   10   15 kilometers

Hoh Indian
Reservation

6 101

7
To Hoquiam

1	Cape Flattery		**5**	Toleak Point
2	Shi Shi Beach and Point of the Arches		**6**	Jefferson Cove
3	Ozette Triangle		**7**	Ruby Beach
4	Rialto Beach and Hole-in-the-Wall			

The Olympic Coast

TRAIL	DIFFICULTY	LENGTH	TYPE	USES & ACCESS	TERRAIN	FLORA & FAUNA	OTHER
1	2	1.4	✏	🚶 🐕 👫		🌲 🐦 🦌	🔭 ⛏
2	3	7.8	✏	🚶 🎒	🏔 ✳		🔭 ⛏
3	3–4	9.0	↻	🚶 🎒	✳	🌲 🦌	🏠
4	2	3.0	✏	🚶 🐕 👫	✳	🐦	⛏
5	4	12.4	✏	🎒	🏔 ❚❚ ✳		🔭
6	3	5.2	✏	🚶	✳	🌲 🐦	
7	1 and 3	5.8	✏	🚶 👫		🐦 🦌	🔭

USES & ACCESS	TYPE	TERRAIN	FLORA & FAUNA	OTHER
🚶 Day Hiking	↻ Loop	🔺 Summit	🌲 Old-Growth Forest	🔭 Viewpoint
🎒 Backpacking	↰ Semi-loop	🏔 Steep	✳ Wildflowers	⛏ Geologic Interest
🚵 Mountain Biking	✏ Out-and-back	🌊 Lake	🐦 Birds	🏠 Historic Interest
🐎 Horses		❚❚ Waterfall	🦌 Wildlife	
👫 Child-Friendly	DIFFICULTY - 1 2 3 4 5 + less more	✳ Tidepool		

The Olympic Coast

Cape Flattery 36

Though not a beach walk, this forest path earns its coastal status from its destination, Cape Flattery, which sits at the far northwestern tip of the Olympic Peninsula and, for that matter, the entire continental United States. This remote and ruggedly beautiful spot features crashing waves, views of large Tatoosh Island, abundant wildlife, enormous sea caves, and dozens of scenic rock formations in a series of deep coves and jutting peninsulas. That's a whole lot of highlights in a short and relatively easy package.

Shi Shi Beach and Point of the Arches 41

Save this stellar hike for good weather and a minus tide (an unusually low tide) to enjoy coastal hiking at its finest. After slogging along an often-muddy trail (wear boots, not tennis shoes), you arrive at what is consistently rated as one of the country's most beautiful beaches. From there you can explore a host of nearby sea arches, tidepools, and photogenic sea stacks. This place will provide memories for a lifetime.

Ozette Triangle 47

One of the most famous and popular longer hikes on the Olympic Coast, the Ozette Triangle earns its fame with a rich assortment of outdoor treasures. Ample wildlife, coastal scenery, beautiful forests, and even some American Indian petroglyphs explain its reputation—all excellent reasons for you to take this fun hike as well.

Rialto Beach and Hole-in-the-Wall ... 55

This easy walk along a sandy beach leads to a dramatic and bulky sea arch, where you have the opportunity to literally walk right through the hole in the arch (at low tide, anyway) to the pretty cove on the other side. Throw in lots of tidepools, a few impressive sea stacks and pinnacles, and practically guaranteed sightings of bald eagles, and you can understand why this beach is so well-liked. This trip isn't for solitude lovers, but just about everyone else will enjoy it immensely.

TRAIL 4

Day hiking, dogs allowed (part of the way), child-friendly
3.0 miles
Out-and-back
Difficulty: 1 **2** 3 4 5

Toleak Point ... 59

Perhaps the finest and most satisfying one-night backpacking trip on the Olympic Coast, this fun outing takes you on an extremely scenic, but sometimes grueling, trek past pocket beaches, hundreds of sea stacks, and countless tidepools. The goal is a collection of idyllic beachside campsites where you can relax and watch the sunset while being lulled to sleep by waves. You also must contend, however, with steep scramble trails over headlands, tide issues, and sometimes-muddy trails, so be prepared.

TRAIL 5

Backpacking
12.4 miles
Out-and-back
Difficulty: 1 2 3 **4** 5

Jefferson Cove ... 66

Solitude seekers will delight in this hidden coastal gem. Simply locate this out-of-the-way trailhead and wait for low tide to scramble over two clusters of very slippery boulders; then experience a dramatically scenic beach and cliff-lined cove. The tidepooling and wildlife-watching are some of the best in the area.

TRAIL 6

Day hiking
5.2 miles
Out-and-back
Difficulty: 1 2 **3** 4 5

Ruby Beach ... 71

The most photographed location on the Olympic Coast, Ruby Beach teems with people during the summer season. By visiting on a weekday in the off-season, you can avoid most of the crowds. In addition, savvy hikers know that solitude is easy to find even in the high season by extending their outing along the long and lonely beach north of famous Abbey Island to the mouth of the Hoh River.

TRAIL 7

Day hiking, child-friendly
Up to 5.8 miles
Out-and-back
Difficulty: **1** 2 3 4 5

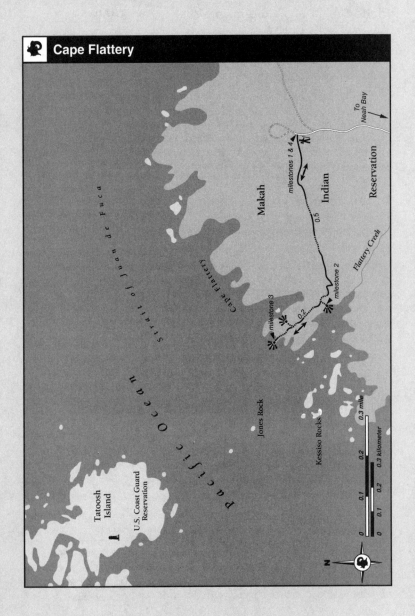

Cape Flattery

Makah

Indian

Reservation

To Neah Bay

milestones 1 & 4

0.5

Flattery Creek

milestone 2

milestone 3

0.2

Cape Flattery

Strait of Juan de Fuca

Pacific Ocean

Tatoosh Island

U.S. Coast Guard Reservation

Jones Rock

Kessiso Rocks

0.3 mile

0   0.1   0.2   0.3 kilometer

0   0.1   0.2

N

Cape Flattery

Cape Flattery protrudes from the very tip of the Olympic Peninsula and forms the northwesternmost point in the Lower 48. Fittingly, visiting this remote location really gives you the impression of being at the end of the world. Waves pound the cliffs and sea caves at your feet, while winds contort the trees and carry off any hats not strapped down carefully enough. The Makah Indians, who own this land, manage the cape as a nature sanctuary, and you can understand why; it's a marvelous location for viewing wildlife, including sea otters, various species of whales, and a host of interesting birds. They could just as easily manage it as a scenic viewpoint, however, as the vistas of islands both near and far, dozens of jagged rock pinnacles, and dramatic cliff-lined coves are exceptional. For such a short and relatively easy hike, the rewards of this outing are hard to beat.

TRAIL USE
Day hiking, dogs allowed (on leash), child-friendly

LENGTH
1.4 miles, 1 hour

CUMULATIVE ELEVATION
200'

DIFFICULTY
- 1 **2** 3 4 5 +

TRAIL TYPE
Out-and-back

SURFACE TYPE
Gravel, boardwalk, dirt

CONTOUR MAP
Custom Correct *North Olympic Coast* or Green Trails *Cape Flattery* #98S

START & END
N48° 23.093'
W124° 42.944'

FEATURES
Abundant wildlife, dramatic views, rugged headlands

FACILITIES
Restrooms

Best Time

The trail is open all year, but it is best saved for a clear day (to enjoy the views) with light winds (wind can blow extremely hard at the cape). Mornings are usually better for photography and wildlife viewing.

Finding the Trail

Drive US 101 about 11.5 miles north of Forks or 43 miles west of Port Angeles to a junction near the tiny village of Sappho at milepost 203.7. Turn north on Washington Highway 113, following signs to Northwest Coast and Ozette Lake, and drive 10.2

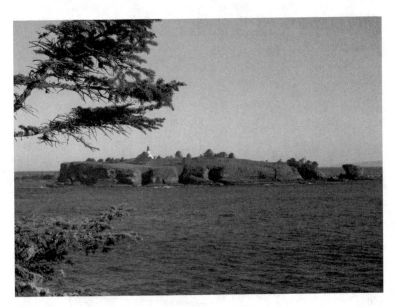

View of Tatoosh Island *from Cape Flattery*

miles to the junction with WA 112. Go straight, now on WA 112, and stay on this slow and winding road for 23.2 miles to the point where you enter the Makah Indian Reservation. Continue on the main road for another 3.1 miles to the community of Neah Bay and Washburn's General Store on your left. Stop here to purchase the required recreational use permit, which allows you to hike on Makah Indian Reservation lands. As of 2014, the charge was a very reasonable $10 for a pass good for the entire calendar year.

Permit in hand, continue west through Neah Bay, staying on the main road for 0.9 mile, and then make two 90-degree turns, first left on Fort Street, and then right on Third Street. Just 0.1 mile after the second 90-degree turn is a junction. Go left on paved Cape Flattery Road and drive 2.4 miles to a junction just before the Makah Tribal Center. Go straight and stay on this winding paved road for another 5.5 miles to the well-marked Cape Trail parking lot.

Trail Description

The wide and exceptionally well-built gravel trail departs from the northwest corner of the parking lot ►1 and descends at a moderately steep grade through an attractive forest of western red cedars, western hemlocks, and Sitka spruces. Sword ferns, salal, and other ground cover species crowd the forest floor. After 0.2 mile, the trail narrows somewhat as it alternates between a gravel or dirt surface and a series of wooden boardwalks. The trail's careful construction by the Makah tribe guarantees that, despite the often-rainy weather, there is very little mud.

Old-Growth Forest

As you near the coastline, the sound of pounding surf becomes increasingly evident and gradually replaces the songs of forest birds and the sound of wind in the trees. The path continues to steadily lose elevation, sometimes in boardwalk stairs and sometimes via thick log cross sections that serve as arboreal stepping-stones. At just under 0.5 mile, a boardwalk side trail goes 30 yards to the left to a wooden platform ►2 with a great view down into a rugged cove that features several scenic islands. Steep cliffs riddled with sea caves surround the cove. Binoculars will come in handy here to observe the colonies of gulls and pelagic cormorants that nest on the islands, or to watch the antics of sea otters, which can usually be seen bobbing in the cove's surf.

Viewpoint

Birds

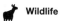
Wildlife

Back on the main trail, you continue to gradually descend on wooden boardwalks past another viewing platform, this one on the right and overlooking a smaller cove on that side of the cape. The trail ends shortly thereafter at a pair of view stands at the cliff-edged tip of the cape. ►3 Don your Windbreaker (the winds often howl here) and watch the waves pound the rocks at your feet as they slowly enlarge the enormous sea caves in the sandstone underneath you. In time, this erosion will cause the ground to collapse and the cape to

Viewpoint

Geologic Interest

Birds

Wildlife

continue its slow retreat in the face of the relentless ocean. In the meantime, you can admire the wildlife, which includes a wide range of birds (puffins, cormorants, scoters, gulls, murres, and eagles, among others), as well as sea otters, sea lions, and possibly whales. If the critters aren't around, there is always the view to enjoy. Tatoosh Island, with its prominent lighthouse, sits only about 0.6 mile offshore and guards the entrance to the Strait of Juan de Fuca. Meanwhile, to the north, the mountains of Canada's Vancouver Island fill the distant skyline. It's a wonderful spot to enjoy the scene before turning back to the parking lot. ▶4

MILESTONES

▶1	0.0	Take Cape Trail from parking lot (N48° 23.093' W124° 42.944')
▶2	0.5	Viewing platform on left (N48° 23.057' W124° 43.501')
▶3	0.7	Tip of Cape Flattery (N48° 23.153' W124° 43.602')
▶4	1.4	Return to parking lot (N48° 23.093' W124° 42.944')

Shi Shi Beach and Point of the Arches

With ideal conditions—sunny skies and a minus tide (an unusually low tide)—there probably isn't a more spectacular coastal hiking destination in the United States than Shi Shi Beach and Point of the Arches. This outstanding trip combines a glorious strip of sand—which despite, or perhaps because of, its remoteness has previously been designated the nation's best nature beach by the Travel Channel—and one of the most impressive collections of rock pinnacles and sea arches in the world. Wildlife, especially birds, is abundant, which explains why all of the countless offshore rocks in this area are protected in the Flattery Rocks National Wildlife Refuge. Add to this the fine tidepooling and surprising solitude, and you have a real winner. The main drawback for this stretch of paradise is a sometimes *very* muddy trail, so leave the tennis shoes in the car and be prepared for mud-splattered pants and boots.

Best Time

The trail is open all year, but it is best saved for a clear day with an extra low tide. Summer and fall are preferred; they typically have *marginally* less mud on the approach trail than the winter and spring months.

Finding the Trail

Drive US 101 about 11.5 miles north of Forks or 43 miles west of Port Angeles to a junction near the tiny village of Sappho at milepost 203.7. Turn

TRAIL USE
Day hiking, backpacking

LENGTH
7.8 miles, 3.5–4 hours (or overnight)

CUMULATIVE ELEVATION
250'

DIFFICULTY
- 1 2 **3** 4 5 +

TRAIL TYPE
Out-and-back

SURFACE TYPE
Gravel, boardwalk, dirt, mud, sand

CONTOUR MAP
Custom Correct *North Olympic Coast*

START & END
N48° 17.616'
W124° 39.890'

FEATURES
Coastal scenery, numerous sea arches, tidepooling, beach

FACILITIES
Restrooms

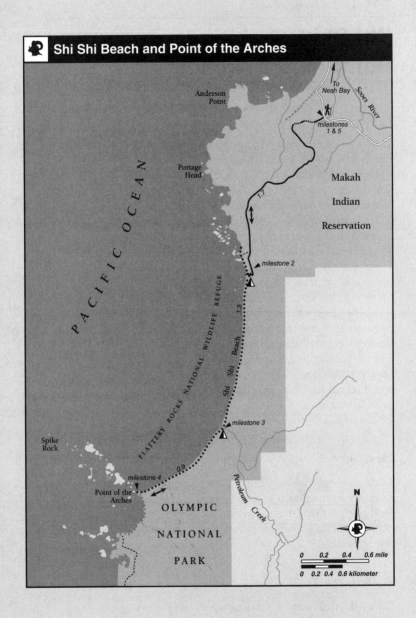

Shi Shi Beach and Point of the Arches

Anderson Point

To Neah Bay

Sooes River

milestones 1 & 5

Portage Head

Makah

Indian

Reservation

1.7

P A C I F I C   O C E A N

milestone 2

1.3

FLATTERY ROCKS NATIONAL WILDLIFE REFUGE

Shi Shi Beach

milestone 3

Spike Rock

0.9

milestone 4

Point of the Arches

OLYMPIC

NATIONAL

PARK

Petroleum Creek

N

0   0.2   0.4   0.6 mile

0   0.2 0.4 0.6 kilometer

north on Washington Highway 113, following signs to Northwest Coast and Ozette Lake, and drive 10.2 miles to the junction with WA 112. Go straight, now on WA 112, and stay on this slow and winding road for 23.2 miles to the point where you enter the Makah Indian Reservation. Continue on the main road for another 3.1 miles to the community of Neah Bay and Washburn's General Store on your left. Stop here to purchase the required recreational use permit, which allows you to hike on Makah Indian Reservation lands. As of 2014, the charge was a very reasonable $10 for a pass good for the entire calendar year.

Permit in hand, continue west through Neah Bay, staying on the main road for 0.9 mile, and then make two 90-degree turns, first left on Fort Street, and then right on Third Street. Just 0.1 mile after the second 90-degree turn is a junction. Go left on paved Cape Flattery Road and drive 2.4 miles to a junction just before the Makah Tribal Center. Follow signs to Hobuck Beach and Fish Hatchery, and turn left on Hobuck Road, immediately crossing a bridge over the Waatch River. After 0.1 mile, go straight at a four-way junction and then stay on the main paved road, always following signs to the fish hatchery, for 4.2 miles to the small, gravel parking lot and trailhead on the right.

Trail Description

The trail goes southwest from the parking lot ▶1 through the usual dense coastal forest dominated by Sitka spruces. The Makah tribe has recently improved the first part of this once notoriously muddy route with gravel and boardwalks, so it is now more of a joy than a slog. The views are restricted by trees, however, so you will wend your way through tunnels of shrubbery and second-growth forest. You will cross wooden bridges and

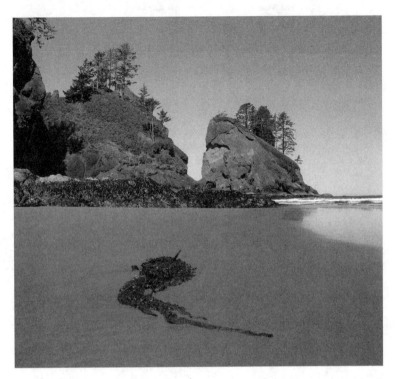

Low tide scene *at Point of the Arches*

make a few minor ups and downs but never change your elevation significantly. The improved trail ends at about 0.75 mile.

At the end of the good trail, you are left to negotiate almost 1 mile of the old trail, with its frequent stretches of deep, dark, gooey mud. This is why boots, rather than tennis shoes, are strongly recommended for this hike. Although muddy, the trail is nearly level as it goes south toward the beach. After about 0.8 mile on this older trail, you'll notice a few short and enticing side paths that go to the right to partially obstructed cliff-top viewpoints of the Pacific Ocean.

Viewpoint

At 1.7 miles, you reach the Olympic National Park boundary ▶2 and a wilderness permit station for overnight hikers. From here, the trail descends a series of short but very steep switchbacks, rapidly

Steep

losing about 150 feet to a pair of fine campsites just before you reach the northern end of magnificent Shi Shi Beach.

This long strip of sand is absolutely idyllic, with big waves, jagged rocks, and some of the best tidepooling in the country. Before heading south to Point of the Arches, take 10 minutes to scramble over the minor headland at the north end of Shi Shi Beach to a gorgeous little cove with a postcard-perfect arch of its own. The tidepools here house an incredible abundance of colorful sea life.

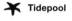 Tidepool

Going south on Shi Shi Beach is extremely scenic but rather tiring because it is difficult to get solid footing in the loose sand. It's hard to complain, however, with coastal scenery this, well, *perfect* is the only word I can come up with. Almost 1.2 miles south of when you first came to the beach are two good campsites on either side of Petroleum Creek. ►**3** Don't worry; the creek's water is not the least bit oily and is perfectly safe to drink after the usual filtering.

From Petroleum Creek, it's another 0.9 mile of hiking on mostly hard-packed sand to the pinnacle-strewn tip of Point of the Arches. ►**4** This marvelous spot is a fantasyland of, yes, sea arches, as well as tidepools, rock towers, islands, and great ocean views. At low tide, plenty of photo taking and exploring is definitely in order. Sadly, all good things must come to an end, with, in this case, time and tide restrictions eventually forcing you to turn around and return to the trailhead ►**5** the way you came. *Tip:* To delay that end for a little while, try turning this into a short backpacking trip with a night (or two) at Petroleum Creek. You won't regret it.

 Tidepool

 Geologic Interest

⋀ MILESTONES

▶1   0.0   Take trail from parking lot (N48° 17.616' W124° 39.890')

▶2   1.7   Enter Olympic National Park just above Shi Shi Beach
(N48° 16.497' W124° 40.702')

▶3   3.0   Petroleum Creek (N48° 15.337' W124° 41.102')

▶4   3.9   Point of the Arches (N48° 14.839' W124° 42.040')

▶5   7.8   Retrace beach route and trail to trailhead
(N48° 17.616' W124° 39.890')

Ozette Triangle

Because coastal trails necessarily tend to follow a narrow, linear landform, it is extremely rare to find a beach hike that forms a loop. The Ozette Triangle is a wonderful exception to that rule. Here, two diverging forest trails connect a superb section of scenic shoreline to form a nearly perfect triangle. But it isn't merely the route's shape on a map that makes this the most famous day hike or weekend backpacking trip on the Olympic Coast. People flock here to enjoy the abundant wildlife (including everything from sea otters to eagles), extensive areas of tidepools, wonderful beach campsites, American Indian petroglyphs, and coastal scenery. The trip includes some rugged hiking along the coastal leg of the triangle, but it is all great fun.

There are no limits on the number of day hikers, but due to the extreme popularity of this trip, the National Park Service has imposed tight restrictions on the number of overnight visitors allowed to stay in this area. May 1–September 30, *all backpackers must obtain a reserved permit* for one of the few available sites. No first-come, first-serve permits are given out. To apply for a reservation, visit the park's website (**nps.gov/olym**), download a Wilderness Camping Permit Reservation Request form, fill out your information and planned itinerary, include your payment, and then send it by snail mail or fax (360-565-3108) to the Wilderness Information Center.

Best Time

The trail is open all year and is good at any time. Summers are quite crowded (especially for

TRAIL USE
Day hiking, backpacking

LENGTH
9.0 miles, 5 hours (or overnight)

CUMULATIVE ELEVATION
360'

DIFFICULTY
- 1 2 **3 4** 5 +
(*depending on tides and time of year*)

TRAIL TYPE
Loop

SURFACE TYPE
Gravel, boardwalk, dirt, sand, rocks

CONTOUR MAP
Custom Correct *North Olympic Coast*

START & END
N48° 09.282'
W124° 40.136'

FEATURES
Diverse coastal scenery, American Indian petroglyphs, tidepooling, coastal forests, abundant wildlife

FACILITIES
Restrooms, water, picnic tables, ranger station

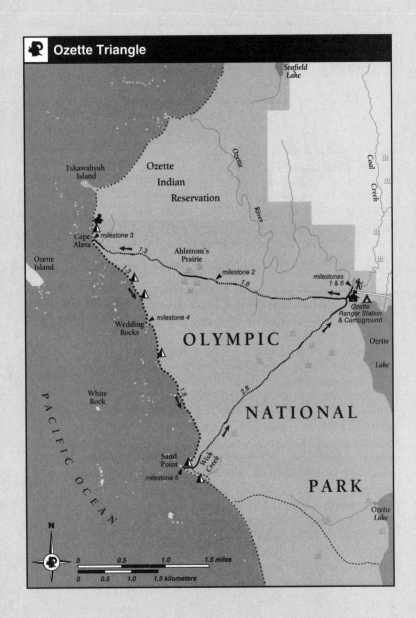

Ozette Triangle

Seafield Lake

Ozette River

Coal Creek

Tskawahyah Island

Ozette Indian Reservation

Cape Alava

milestone 3

1.9

Ahlstrom's Prairie

milestone 2

1.8

milestones 1 & 6

Ozette Island

1.3

Ozette Ranger Station & Campground

milestone 4

Wedding Rocks

OLYMPIC

Ozette Lake

White Rock

1.8

2.8

NATIONAL

P A C I F I C   O C E A N

Sand Point

Wish Creek

milestone 5

PARK

Ozette Lake

N

0   0.5   1.0   1.5 miles

0   0.5   1.0   1.5 kilometers

backpackers), and winter storms may wash away some beaches or topple numerous trees across the narrow shoreline, making for strenuous hiking. Thus, spring and fall are probably the best times to visit. Low tide makes hiking the coastal section much easier and more interesting.

Finding the Trail

Drive US 101 about 11.5 miles north of Forks or 43 miles west of Port Angeles to a junction near the tiny village of Sappho at milepost 203.7. Turn north on Washington Highway 113, following signs to Northwest Coast and Ozette Lake, and drive 10.2 miles to the junction with WA 112. Go straight, now on WA 112, and proceed 11 miles to a prominent junction with the Hoko–Ozette Road near milepost 12.5.

Turn left (south), following signs to Ozette Lake and Coastal Trails. Drive this slow and winding paved road for 21.8 miles to its end at a large gravel turnaround and trailhead parking area immediately past the small, seasonally staffed Ozette Ranger Station. This trailhead comes just 0.2 mile after you pass the turnoff to the Ozette Lake Campground, a convenient and comfortable place to spend the night if you are starting your hike early the next morning.

Trail Description

The trail begins at the south end of the parking lot ▶1 beside a large signboard. The gravel path very quickly crosses a bridge over sluggish Coal Creek, goes past the back side of Ozette Ranger Station, and then takes a larger bridge over the Ozette River, the clear-flowing outlet to nearby Ozette Lake. The heavily used path then climbs a bit through a forest of red alders, Sitka spruces, Douglas-firs, and western red cedars. Beneath these tall specimens are the usual dense understory and ground cover, including a particular abundance of salmonberry, deer and sword ferns, and false lilies of the valley. At a little more than 0.1 mile, the trail splits at the start of the loop. Either direction is equally good. The route is described here counterclockwise, which means you should turn right toward Cape Alava.

The trail now works its way through a virtual tunnel of coastal shrubs and trees with lots of salal, salmonberry, and evergreen huckleberry. In wetter places, you will also see plenty of skunk cabbage. After 0.3 mile, you encounter the first of what will add up to several miles of boardwalk trail. These boardwalks are in place to reduce the problems of mud and erosion in this soggy climate, and they work well for that purpose. When it rains, however, the wooden boardwalks can be quite slippery, so please watch your step. (*Tip:* Soft-soled sneakers or other shoes offer better footing than lug-soled boots.) In a few places, the old wooden boardwalk has been replaced with a conglomerate plastic material, which lasts longer and affords better footing but doesn't look very natural. In between the long boardwalk sections, the trail is mostly gravel. Both surfaces include countless little stairsteps that guide you over the rolling terrain.

At not quite 1.8 miles, you come to Ahlstrom's Prairie, ▶2 a large opening in the forest with lots of brush and thick, wiry grasses. This was once the site of a homestead for a Swedish immigrant, but it has long since reverted to wildland. After passing through the prairie, the trail reenters dense forest and then offers up another 0.5 mile or so of viewless, but pleasant, up-and-down hiking.

By about 2.5 miles, the sound of the surf becomes an increasingly prominent part of your hiking experience. Soon thereafter, you negotiate a series of irregularly spaced downhill steps in the

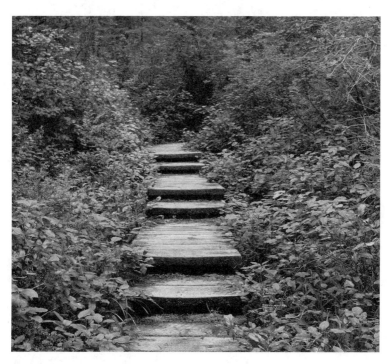

Typical section *of boardwalk to Cape Alava*

boardwalk. Finally, a short downhill on dirt trail leads to the rocky shoreline at Cape Alava. ►3

Large and forest-covered Ozette Island sits off to the west–southwest, while much smaller Tskawahyah Island can be seen to the north. At very low tide, a shallow zone of tidepools and seaweed-covered rocks extends several hundred yards out into the ocean, almost reaching Ozette Island. This rocky area is great for exploring if you watch your step and keep a careful eye on the tides. At any tide, and in any season, wildlife is extremely abundant around Cape Alava. You can expect to see lots of seals, sea lions (listen for their croaking barks), sea otters, raccoons, deer, ravens, bald eagles, black oystercatchers, and much more. To

 Tidepool

 Wildlife

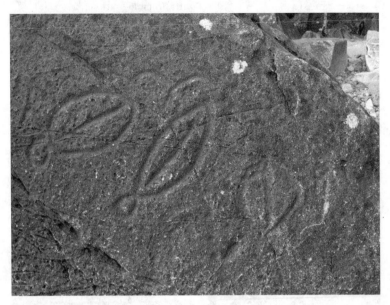

Fish petroglyphs *at Wedding Rocks*

find the designated camping area and seasonal Cape
Alava Ranger Station, follow either the inland path
or the rugged shoreline north for about 0.3 mile. If
you have the time, the beach north of Cape Alava
is well worth exploring. The route in that direction
soon crosses into the Ozette Indian Reservation, so
inland travel is prohibited, but the beach is open to
all hikers. If you go here, however, please do not
hike out to Tskawahyah Island, which is connected
to the shore by a peninsula of sand, because this site
is sacred to American Indians.

The recommended loop hike goes south from
Cape Alava. It is a scenic but rugged route with
lots of downed trees to climb over or (when the
tide is lower) walk around. There are also plenty of
treacherously loose and slippery rocks to deal with,
so watch your step. Thus, while the hiking is enormously fun and has almost no elevation gain or loss,
it is not an easy walk on the beach.

Between 0.8 and 1.1 miles south of Cape Alava, you pass a series of small but inviting campsites. Unfortunately, fresh water is usually not available here, so you'll have to carry in your own. At 1.3 miles from Cape Alava, you will come across a minor rocky protuberance called the Wedding Rocks. ►4 Spend some time in this area to seek out the sometimes-hard-to-find petroglyphs that are carved into several of the large, dark-colored boulders. With patience and a little exploring, you will find representations of fish, whales, dogs, and other animals, as well as sailing ships. It is much easier to explore and crawl around these huge boulders when the tide is lower. If the tide is high, you may be forced to skirt the Wedding Rocks via a short inland scramble trail.

Historic Interest

At the next little promontory, not quite 0.4 mile south of Wedding Rocks, is another good but waterless campsite directly across from a rock pinnacle with a tiny sea arch in it.

Sand Point ►5 comes along at 3.1 miles south of Cape Alava. This headland curves out into the ocean, reaching its end at a grass-covered bump. Though a marked trail goes inland before you reach the end of Sand Point, you may wish to continue forward to explore the tip and enjoy the tidepooling and fine views up and down this wild coast. Amid the forest, inland from the point, are dozens of excellent campsites. Water is available from tiny Wish Creek on the south side of the point. If you want to spend more time on the coast, invest that time on the lovely 2-mile strip of sand stretching south from Sand Point. It is one of the prettiest wilderness beaches on the Olympic Coast.

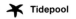

Tidepool

To find the trail back to Ozette Lake, work your way a short distance inland, past great campsites and on use trails that pass through head-high tangles of salal bushes, to the main marked trail. Here, you turn left, following occasional signs to Ozette Ranger Station.

Except for the lack of anything like Ahlstrom's Prairie, the trail back from Sand Point is much like the trail out to Cape Alava in reverse. The partly gravel but mostly boardwalk path stays in forest as it climbs a bit away from the pounding surf, and it then goes gradually up and down in stairsteps all the way back to the junction near Ozette Lake. Keep right and retrace the last 0.1 mile to the trailhead. ▶6

		MILESTONES
▶1	0.0	Take trail from parking lot (N48° 09.282' W124° 40.136')
▶2	1.8	Enter Ahlstrom's Prairie (N48° 09.342' W124° 42.263')
▶3	3.1	Cape Alava (N48° 09.647' W124° 43.896')
▶4	4.4	Wedding Rocks (N48° 08.951' W124° 43.216')
▶5	6.2	Sand Point (N48° 07.554' W124° 42.688')
▶6	9.0	Return to trailhead (N48° 09.282' W124° 40.136')

Rialto Beach and Hole-in-the-Wall

Rialto Beach is, understandably, one of the most popular stretches of sand in Washington State. The wide and photogenic beach offers excellent wildlife viewing (especially for bald eagles) and beautiful vistas of the vast Pacific Ocean and some scenic nearby islands and pinnacles. It also has easy access via a good paved road. Unlike most other Olympic Coast beaches, you can even bring your dog and let him or her play in the sand. All of this means that solitude seekers probably should head elsewhere, unless they have the ability to visit in the off-season on a weekday. But the rewards of hiking here are many, especially for those who want to visit and even, at low tide, walk *through* a massive sea arch. It is well worth the relatively short hike and the constant company of other admiring people.

Best Time

The beach is open all year, but it is much better with a low tide and, for greater seclusion, on a weekday during the off-season.

Finding the Trail

Drive US 101 about 1 mile north of Forks to a junction with Washington Highway 110 (also known as La Push Road) near milepost 193.1. Turn left (west), following signs for La Push and Mora. Drive 8 miles, and then turn right onto Mora Road. You enter Olympic National Park after 2.8 miles, and then continue another 2.2 miles to the road-end day-use parking lot for Rialto Beach.

TRAIL USE
Day hiking, dogs allowed (south of Ellen Creek), child-friendly

LENGTH
3.0 miles, 1.5–2 hours

CUMULATIVE ELEVATION
less than 10'

DIFFICULTY
- 1 **2** 3 4 5 +

TRAIL TYPE
Out-and-back

SURFACE TYPE
Sand

CONTOUR MAP
Custom Correct *North Olympic Coast* or Green Trails *Ozette* #130S

START & END
N47° 55.285'
W124° 38.285'

FEATURES
Long beach, large sea arch, bald eagles, tidepools

FACILITIES
Restrooms, picnic area, water, trash can

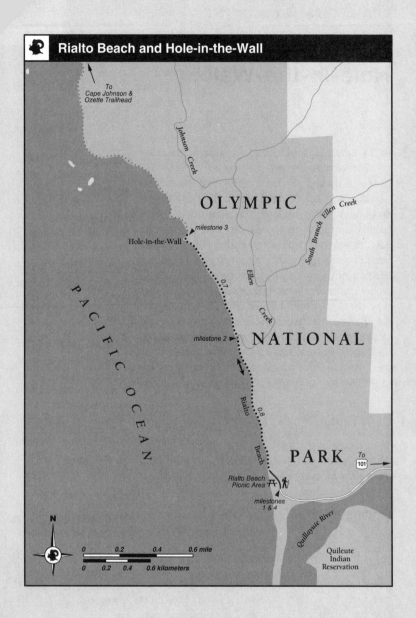

Rialto Beach and Hole-in-the-Wall

To Cape Johnson &
Ozette Trailhead

Johnson Creek

OLYMPIC

milestone 3

Hole-in-the-Wall

0.7

South Branch Ellen Creek

Ellen

Creek

milestone 2

NATIONAL

Rialto

0.8

Beach

PACIFIC OCEAN

PARK

To
101

Rialto Beach
Picnic Area

milestones
1 & 4

Quillayute River

Quileute
Indian
Reservation

N

| 0 | 0.2 | 0.4 | 0.6 mile |

| 0 | 0.2 | 0.4 | 0.6 kilometers |

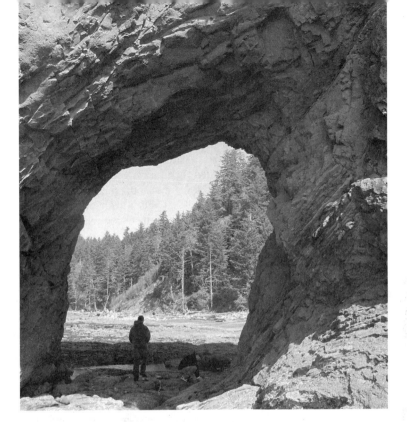

Hiker walking *through arch at Hole-in-the-Wall*

Trail Description

Walk north from the parking lot ▶1 on a trail that goes past a developed picnic area at the edge of the forest. After about 100 yards, you emerge from the trees onto the gray sands of long and lovely Rialto Beach. The sand of this very popular beach is often loose pebbles, so the walking can be a bit tiring, but it is also very rewarding, with nice views southwest to James Island, north to Cape Johnson, and immediately beside you to countless low, jagged rocks and tidepools. On the land side of the beach are numerous dead snags killed by the salt spray and the ever-advancing surf. Bald eagles often perch on these snags.

 Tidepool

 Birds

At 0.8 mile, Ellen Creek ►2 crosses the beach, usually necessitating a simple ankle-deep wade. Dogs are not allowed on Rialto Beach north of this creek.

The next highlight arrives just 0.6 mile later when you pass a particularly photogenic pair of tall, sharply pointed rock pinnacles that rise out of the beach. Just a bit more than 0.1 mile after these pinnacles is Hole-in-the-Wall. ►3 At low tide, hikers can walk across some mussel-covered rocks to the arch's enormous hole and then simply walk through to reach the beach on the other side. At high tide, when the hole in the arch is inaccessible, you'll have to use a steep scramble trail that climbs over the inland side of the rock. *Tip:* Late in the afternoon, photographers will want to use the inland route, regardless of the tides, to take advantage of the excellent late-day lighting looking back to the south along pinnacle-strewn Rialto Beach.

Geologic Interest ✦

The cove north of Hole-in-the-Wall is scenic and well worth exploring. If you are feeling ambitious, you can continue hiking another 2.2 miles to the rocky base of Cape Johnson. Going around that cape and beyond requires backpacking; you must pay careful attention to the tides if you choose to go this way. Once you've had your fill of exploring, retrace the beach route back to the parking lot. ►4

🚶	**MILESTONES**	
►1	0.0	Take trail from parking lot (N47° 55.285' W124° 38.285')
►2	0.8	Ellen Creek (N47° 55.980' W124° 38.622')
►3	1.5	Hole-in-the-Wall (N47° 56.505' W124° 39.066')
►4	3.0	Return to parking lot (N47° 55.285' W124° 38.285')

Toleak Point

Arguably the best one-night backpacking trip on the Olympic Coast, this challenging but rewarding trip offers plenty of variety for hikers. Included along the way is everything that makes this strip of wilderness coast so unique and beautiful: abundant wildlife, colorful tidepool creatures, terrific sunsets, rugged headlands, wild beaches, dramatic rock formations, and outstanding beach campsites far from any roads. Like all longer overnight trips on the Olympic Coast, it also requires some challenging hiking. You'll be forced to take rugged inland scramble trails over Taylor Point and (depending on the tide) Scotts Bluff that include some ridiculously steep grades where ropes are installed to help you *pull* yourself up the cliff face. There are also plenty of muddy sections, roots to avoid, and a couple of headlands without inland trails, where you will have to wait for a medium to low tide to get around. But if you are able and willing, you'll be rewarded with a coastal backpacking experience that is second to none.

Best Time

The trail and beach route are open all year, but the beaches may get washed out by winter storms, and the mud on inland trails has been known to swallow small children during the rainy season (just kidding, but only a little). It is better, therefore, to hike this route May–October. You will need a low to medium tide to get around a couple of points south of Scott Creek.

TRAIL USE
Backpacking

LENGTH
12.4 miles, 2 days

CUMULATIVE ELEVATION
950'

DIFFICULTY
- 1 2 3 **4** 5 +

TRAIL TYPE
Out-and-back

SURFACE TYPE
Sand, dirt, mud

CONTOUR MAP
Custom Correct *South Olympic Coast* or Green Trails *La Push* #163S

START & END
N47° 53.428'
W124° 35.955'

FEATURES
Wilderness beaches, rugged headlands, great sunsets, tidepools, wildlife, dramatic coastal scenery

FACILITIES
Restrooms

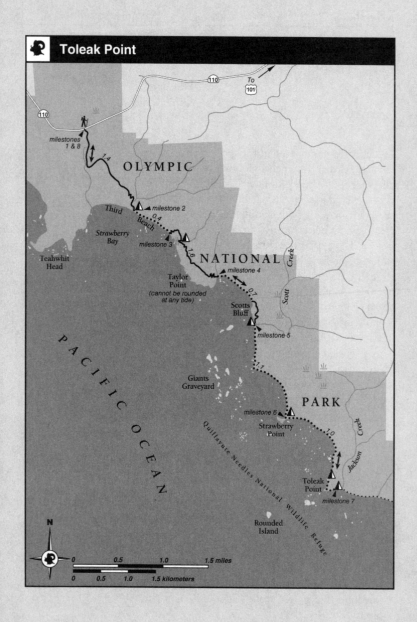

Toleak Point

110

To 101

milestones 1 & 8

OLYMPIC

14

Third Beach

milestone 2

0.4

Strawberry Bay

milestone 3

1.6

Teahwhit Head

NATIONAL

Taylor Point
(cannot be rounded
at any tide)

milestone 4

0.7

Scott Creek

Scotts Bluff

milestone 5

PACIFIC OCEAN

Giants Graveyard

1.7

PARK

milestone 6

Strawberry Point

1.0

Jackson Creek

Quillayute Needles National Wildlife Refuge

Toleak Point

milestone 7

Rounded Island

N

0   0.5   1.0   1.5 miles

0   0.5   1.0   1.5 kilometers

Finding the Trail

Drive US 101 about 1 mile north of Forks to a junction near milepost 193.1 with Washington Highway 110 (also known as La Push Road). Turn west, following signs for La Push and Mora, and drive 8 miles to a junction. Go straight, still on La Push Road, and proceed 3.9 miles to the signed Third Beach Trailhead on the left.

Trail Description

The wide gravel trail leads south from the trailhead ▶1 through a relatively open forest of western hemlocks and Sitka spruces. Initially the chattering of Douglas squirrels and the wildly rollicking songs of winter wrens are the dominant sounds, but as you approach the shore, these are gradually replaced by the roar of waves crashing against rocks or breaking on the sand. The gentle and shady forest walk continues for about 1.2 miles to a short downhill that takes you to a nice camping area on Third Beach ▶2 beside a small creek. This lovely sandy beach, which forms the shoreline of Strawberry Bay, is hemmed in by the cliffs of Teahwhit Head to the west and the imposing headland and pinnacles of Taylor Point to the southeast.

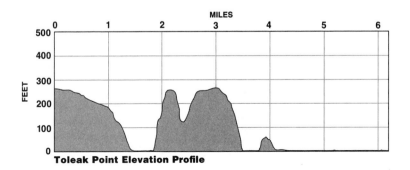

Toleak Point Elevation Profile

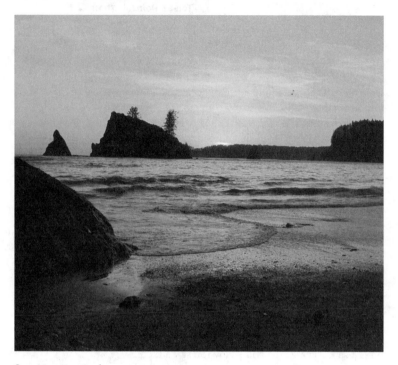

Sunset *at Scott Creek*

Turn left and make your way down the beach toward Taylor Point. Waves crash, gulls squawk, and views abound—in other words, this beach offers all the usual great fun of the wild Olympic Coast. After 0.4 mile, Third Beach ends ▶3 just before you reach a tall waterfall that drops off the cliffs into the surf. This is a fine turnaround point for a short day hike.

Waterfall

Hikers continuing on the recommended backpacking trip should backtrack about 100 yards from the waterfall and look for a sometimes hard-to-see rope ladder going up the steep slope. This is the way to the inland scramble route over otherwise impassable Taylor Point. The rope is installed to help hikers steady themselves and to allow you to literally *pull* yourself up the steep slope. *Tip:* If

Steep

you have a walking stick(s), stow it away before you climb because you will need both hands to hang on to the rope.

The next 0.25 mile is a dirt trail with some sections that are so *extremely* steep that you will be forced to use ropes and rickety ladders to aid your climb. It is a bit of a struggle but surprisingly fun and rewarding, with at least one excellent view of Third Beach and Teahwhit Head along the way. After gaining about 250 feet, the trail abruptly eases off and travels with only minor ups and downs through a dense forest of Sitka spruce. Protruding roots and gooey mud are often present along this route, but that's not a big problem for folks who are now full of confidence after successfully completing the stiff climb. You soon pass a mediocre campsite and then go downhill, losing almost 100 feet, to reach a better campsite beside the tiny creek that feeds the waterfall you observed from Third Beach.

 Viewpoint

The trail quickly regains its recently lost elevation and then winds its way through forest, frequently forcing you to either circumvent or slog through deep mudholes along the way. Eventually the trail descends a series of wooden ladders interspersed with dirt tread to a lovely little pocket beach. ▶4 This beach is graced with a rock pinnacle that has a hardy spruce tree on top of it. The tiny rocky headland on the left (southeast) side of this cove can be rounded at low to medium tide, or you can take a very short scramble trail over its inland side at high tide.

Once past this little headland, you are rewarded with a lovely curving stretch of rocks and hard-packed sand that offers fine vistas out to a distant cluster of tall pinnacles known as the Giants Graveyard. Unfortunately, the easy beach walk only lasts for 0.4 mile when you reach the jumbled boulders and cliffs at the base of Scotts Bluff. At low tide, you can round this point by scrambling over and around a group of large and slippery boulders. At anything other than low tide, however, you will be forced to take the inland scramble trail. The trail starts about 75 yards from the end of the beach, and, as before, it involves a super steep rope pull up the crumbly slopes. Like the trail over Taylor Point, the path around Scotts Bluff has some muddy areas, but it is less of a problem here than on the longer route over Taylor Point. On the south side of Scotts Bluff is a very nice camping area beside Scott Creek. ▶5

Steep 🏔️

Walk down the beach south of Scott Creek for 0.5 mile to its end, where a point requires a moderately low tide to round. Beyond this, the scenery remains wild and spectacular as you marvel at tidepools and gape at eroded rock pinnacles and arches, both nearby and far offshore. Another long, curving beach of mostly hard-packed sand takes you to the low headland of Strawberry Point. ▶6 This spot can be rounded at anything but very high tide and is graced with a bulky rock pinnacle covered with shrubbery. On the inland side of Strawberry Point is a nice possible campsite, though there is no reliable source of fresh water nearby.

Tidepool ✖

The next long, curving beach goes for about 1 mile, past a distinctive pyramid-shaped pinnacle, to Toleak Point. ▶7 An extensive area of tidepools at the tip and on the south side of this headland allows for unlimited exploring opportunities during low tide. The point is also extremely scenic, with a nearby wooded island, crashing waves, lovely sand, and rock pinnacles. It's hard to imagine a nicer location for wilderness beach camping, and there are numerous good to outstanding sites available to accommodate this desire. Jackson Creek, on the south side of the point, provides reliable fresh water (filter it first). Enjoy an evening of exploring, a wonderful sunset, and a restful night listening to waves before packing up and returning to the trailhead. ▶8

Tidepool ✖

Note: For even more great coastal scenery, consider continuing south from Toleak Point on the
long, one-way adventure to the Oil City Trailhead
on the Hoh River (17 miles from the Third Beach
Trailhead). This route offers even greater chal-
lenges than the northern approach to Toleak Point,
with even muddier inland trails, lots of scrambling
over slippery rocks, and three creek crossings that
may be impossible after heavy rains. It is well
worth the effort, however, for the prepared and
athletic hiker. A car shuttle is required (see Trail 6
for driving directions).

🚶	**MILESTONES**	
▶1	0.0	Take trail from parking lot (N47° 53.428' W124° 35.955')
▶2	1.4	Campsite on Third Beach (N47° 52.698' W124° 35.265')
▶3	1.8	South end of Third Beach and start of trail over Taylor Point (N47° 52.504' W124° 34.789')
▶4	3.4	Pocket beach on south side of Taylor Point (N47° 52.058' W124° 34.067')
▶5	4.1	Scott Creek (N47° 51.591' W124° 33.467')
▶6	5.2	Strawberry Point (N47° 50.756' W124° 33.013')
▶7	6.2	Toleak Point (N47° 50.068' W124° 32.454')
▶8	12.4	Return to trailhead (N47° 53.428' W124° 35.955')

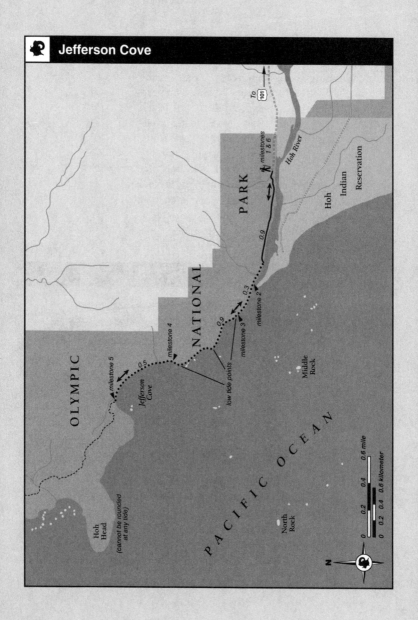

Jefferson Cove

milestones 1 & 6

Hoh River

Hoh Indian Reservation

PARK

NATIONAL

OLYMPIC

0.9

0.3

milestone 2

milestone 3

0.9

milestone 4

low tide points

0.5

milestone 5

Jefferson Cove

Middle Rock

PACIFIC OCEAN

North Rock

Hoh Head (cannot be rounded at any tide)

To 101

0   0.2   0.4   0.6 mile

0   0.2   0.4   0.6 kilometer

N

Jefferson Cove

Jefferson Cove offers the chance to escape the crowds found at some other Olympic Coast destinations (notably Kalaloch Beach, Ruby Beach, and Rialto Beach) without sacrificing anything in the way of scenery. The trail here is a bit off the beaten track, and the beach route requires some tricky low-tide scrambling over unstable and slippery boulders, but for lovers of tidepools and wild coastal scenery, that is a small price to pay.

Best Time

The trail and beach route are open all year. You will need a low tide to get around a couple of headlands south of Jefferson Cove, and low tide is also needed to enjoy the excellent tidepools in the cove.

Finding the Trail

Drive US 101 about 13 miles south of Forks to a junction with Oil City Road near milepost 177.3. Turn right (west), following signs to Cottonwood Recreation Area, and drive west on a road that alternates, at seemingly random intervals, between pavement and good gravel. After 2.4 miles, go straight at the turnoff for Cottonwood Campground and proceed another 2.7 miles to the end of the intermittent pavement. One mile later, bear left at an unsigned fork (the right branch is a heavily used logging road that may or may not be closed off by a gate) and then drive another 4.3 miles to the boundary of Olympic National Park. Just 0.2 mile later is

TRAIL USE
Day hiking

LENGTH
5.2 miles, 2–3 hours

CUMULATIVE ELEVATION
50'

DIFFICULTY
- 1 2 **3** 4 5 +

TRAIL TYPE
Out-and-back

SURFACE TYPE
Dirt, sand, slippery boulders

CONTOUR MAP
Custom Correct *South Olympic Coast* or Green Trails *La Push* #163S

START & END
N47° 44.965'
W124° 25.164'

FEATURES
Solitude, tidepools, dramatic coastal scenery, wildlife

FACILITIES
Restrooms

the road-end turnaround and trailhead, which has parking for about six or seven vehicles.

Trail Description

Old-Growth Forest

The trail to the ocean goes west from the end of the road ►1 amid a dense forest of Sitka spruce and western hemlock. Beneath this tall canopy is a tangled understory of salmonberry, various ferns, and skunk cabbage, among other species. The sometimes muddy path closely follows the steady flow of the milky Hoh River, which is often only a few feet on your left. After 0.75 mile, you leave the rain forest and reach the open, rocky riverbank.

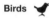
Birds

Look for bald eagles perched on snags beside the river or flying overhead, shopping for a fishy meal.

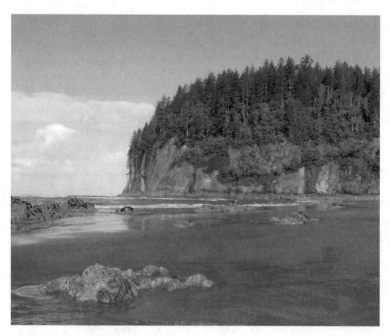

Low tide *scenery at Jefferson Cove*

With the ocean now in sight (and its crashing waves certainly within sound), you follow the riverbank for about 0.15 mile to the beach immediately on the north side of the mouth of the Hoh River. ▶2 Access to the shoreline is usually blocked by a tangled jumble of drift logs that have floated down the Hoh River. Destruction Island and its distinctive lighthouse are visible about 3.5 miles offshore, while a couple of smaller offshore rocky islands and pinnacles are much closer to the beach and a bit to the north.

After carefully making your way over and around all the drift logs to the sand, you turn right (north) and start walking toward the distant jutting point called Hoh Head. The sandy beach soon ends, leaving you to scramble over unstable and slippery boulders as you round a minor headland. ▶3 A low to medium tide is required to make it around this headland. Even at low tide, though, this section requires caution and a fair degree of athleticism to avoid falls or turned ankles. Be sure to check the stability of all boulders before stepping on them, and be especially careful when the rocks are wet or have seaweed on them.

Somewhat easier hiking resumes on the north side of this first headland with a mix of rocks and hard-packed sand. The scenery also improves as you enjoy unobstructed views of impressive Hoh Head with its tall cliffs jutting out into the ocean. Unfortunately, another even longer and more challenging section of slippery rocks soon makes life difficult again. As before, a low to medium tide is required to make this traverse of two adjoining points. The reward comes when you reach the lovely curving sand of the beach in Jefferson Cove. ▶4

The "sand" in Jefferson Cove is actually more akin to loose pebbles, so the surface is tiring to walk on, but unlike the slippery rocks you just crawled over, it is perfectly safe. It is also wildly scenic,

Tidepool ✈

especially as you look north to the cliffs of a nearby (but unnamed) headland bordering the north side of the cove. At low tide, the cove offers wonderful tidepooling.

The beach ends ►5 when you reach the base of the headland's impassable cliffs. For day hikers, this is the place to turn around because the only way forward is to scramble up the rocks and steep cliffs on the inland side of the headland by use of a precarious hanging rope and ladder. It's a tough climb and one that is best left to athletic backpackers doing the very scenic 17-mile overnight traverse to Toleak Point and the Third Beach Trailhead (see Trail 5). Everyone else should simply enjoy the delights of Jefferson Cove and then return to the trailhead. ►6 *Note:* Be sure to check the tide tables and start your return journey well before high tide blocks your retreat to the car.

🚶 MILESTONES

►1	0.0	Take trail from parking lot (N47° 44.965' W124° 25.164')
►2	0.9	Reach the beach at the mouth of the Hoh River (N47° 45.098' W124° 26.291')
►3	1.2	First minor headland (N47° 45.328' W124° 26.817')
►4	2.1	South end of beach in Jefferson Cove (N47° 45.619' W124° 27.023')
►5	2.6	North end of beach in Jefferson Cove (N47° 46.021' W124° 27.408')
►6	5.2	Return to trailhead (N47° 44.965' W124° 25.164')

Ruby Beach

Ruby Beach is a well-known location often depicted on postcards, calendars, and posters. One reason for this fame is that the beach is exceptionally photogenic, with dramatic rock pinnacles and islands. The beach is also extremely easy to reach, with a simple, downhill, 0.2-mile path to the shore. Both of these attributes make it a great destination for hikers as well as photographers. Not surprisingly, easy access and remarkable scenery ensure that the first part of the trip is far from a wilderness experience. On a typical summer day, hundreds of people come to visit this lovely spot. If you want to avoid the crowds, come on a weekday in the off-season, or simply leave the tourists behind by wading across Cedar Creek and walking the long and usually lonely beach north to Hoh River.

Best Time

The trail and beach route are open all year. A low tide will make the hike a bit easier with less soft sand to negotiate. Crossing unbridged Cedar Creek may be difficult after heavy winter rains, so wait a day or two after a significant rainfall. For photographers, low tide provides the best conditions, especially if that tide coincides with sunset, a daily spectacle that is often outstanding at Ruby Beach (weather permitting).

Finding the Trail

Drive US 101 about 25.5 miles south of Forks or 77 miles north of Hoquiam to the well-signed

TRAIL USE
Day hiking,
child-friendly

LENGTH
0.8 mile (to Abbey
Island), 0.5 hour;
5.8 miles to Hoh River,
3 hours

**CUMULATIVE
ELEVATION**
100'

DIFFICULTY
- 1 **2 3** 4 5 +

TRAIL TYPE
Out-and-back

SURFACE TYPE
Gravel, sand

CONTOUR MAP
Custom Correct *South
Olympic Coast* or
Green Trails *La Push*
#163S

START & END
N47° 42.598'
W124° 24.813'

FEATURES
Photogenic beach, dramatic coastal scenery, wildlife, great sunsets

FACILITIES
Restrooms, picnic area

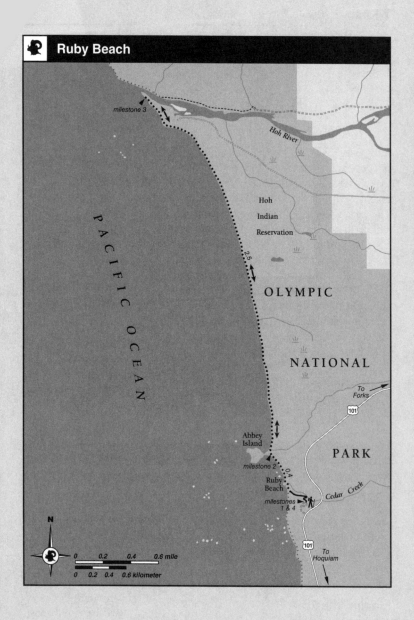

milestone 3

Hoh River

Hoh

Indian

Reservation

2.5

PACIFIC OCEAN

OLYMPIC

NATIONAL

To
Forks

101

Abbey
Island

PARK

milestone 2

0.4

Ruby
Beach

Cedar Creek

*milestones
1 & 4*

N

0   0.2   0.4   0.6 mile

0   0.2   0.4   0.6 kilometer

101

To
Hoquiam

junction with Ruby Beach Road near milepost 164.8. Turn west and drive 0.2 mile to the large gravel parking lot and trailhead.

Trail Description

From the north end of the parking lot, ►1 the trail descends a series of gravel stairsteps through tall brush and open forest. Frequent openings in the forest offer fine views down to Ruby Beach and its famous rock pinnacles and islands. Birdsong is everywhere: the buzz of hummingbirds, the rollicking trill of sparrows, the high-pitched staccato calls of black oystercatchers, and the deep croaks of ravens.

After not quite 0.2 mile, the trail ends at rubble-and drift log–strewn Ruby Beach. It's a lovely and well-known scene, as visitors may recall seeing postcards of the beach's rock towers and islands rising above the perfect little stretch of sand. To add more interest, the first major on-beach pinnacle immediately to your right has two small arches in it.

Turn right (north), walking past the double arch rock, and almost immediately ford Cedar Creek. This chilly stream may temporarily be a challenge to cross after heavy rains, but it is typically only a little more than ankle deep. Almost immediately on the other side of Cedar Creek you come upon Ruby Beach's iconic Abbey Island, ►2 a fortress-shaped monolith topped with shrubs and wind-stunted spruce trees that is reachable at low tide. Other nearby rock pinnacles add to the photogenic qualities of this sight.

If you want solitude, it's surprisingly easy to find because, north of famous Abbey Island, you soon leave the crowds behind as you follow a wide and beautiful strip of sand. On your right (east), a tall, eroded cliff rises from the beach to the forest beyond, while several miles straight ahead you can see the tall cliffs of Hoh Head. The beach is mostly sand but also includes a couple of rocky areas that at extra low tide provide decent tidepooling opportunities. At some unsigned point a little more than a mile north of Abbey Island, you leave Olympic National Park and enter the Hoh Indian Reservation. The tribe graciously allows hikers access to the beach, however, so there's no need to turn around. At 2.7 miles, you come near the end of a road a little before the mouth of the Hoh River, so you may see cars or other people in this area. The now-rocky beach ends after another 0.2 mile at a peninsula on the south side of the mouth of the Hoh River. ▶3 Bald eagles can often be seen flying over the river here, and you may also observe salmon swimming upstream in the cold, milky waters. It's a fitting spot to stop and admire nature before you turn back and return to the trailhead parking lot ▶4 the way you came.

Birds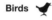

Wildlife

🚶	**MILESTONES**	
▶1	0.0	Take trail from parking lot (N47° 42.593' W124° 24.803')
▶2	0.4	Beach directly opposite Abbey Island (N47° 42.892' W124° 25.125')
▶3	2.9	End of beach on south side of Hoh River (N47° 44.978' W124° 26.130')
▶4	5.8	Return to parking lot (N47° 42.593' W124° 24.803')

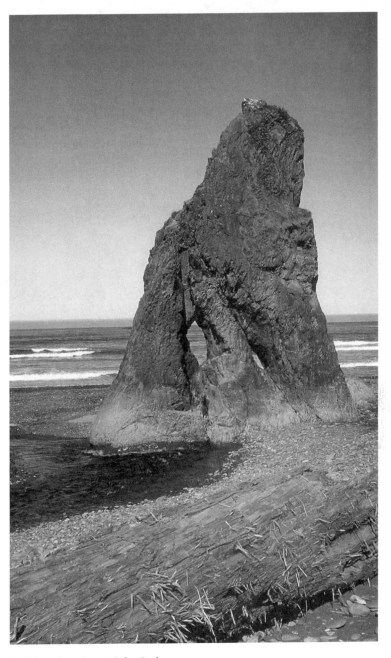

Double arch rock *near Cedar Creek*

West Region: The Rain Forests

West Region:
The Rain Forests

Get ready for *green*, folks, because you are about to enter the world capital for that particularly enchanting color. The forests on the west side of the Olympic Peninsula are drowned in up to 14 feet(!) of rain per year, and the water-loving vegetation of the region has responded with luxuriant growth. In fact, there is so much plant material here that it is positively overwhelming. Towering evergreens reach for the sky. Tangled deciduous trees branch out in the understory. Lichens cover the tree trunks, and thick club mosses drape off every limb. Shrubs, ferns, and a host of other small plants crowd the forest floor. I would say that you get the picture, except that you really don't. You just can't get the true picture without seeing it for yourself.

The waterlogged land beneath all that greenery is ruggedly beautiful in its own right. Peaks and ridges, draped with forests on their lower slopes, rise to great heights here, in fact to the greatest heights on the Olympic Peninsula at 7,980-foot Mount Olympus. And because, with the added elevation, much of the precipitation falls as snow, large glaciers have formed on these peaks, making them shine like jewels when the clouds finally clear. And, believe it or not, those clouds do sometimes clear, especially in mid- to late summer when this land gets its most reliably "good" weather and hiking the high-country trails is at its best.

The low country, amid all those trees, however, is probably best in the off-season. Oh, sure, you might get wet. But, then again, there is always the off chance that you won't, and even when you do, it's not the worst thing in the world. After all, the big trees will protect you from the worst of the rain and wind, and the added moisture makes the forest more attractive as the greens take on a special iridescent quality that is hard to describe but beautiful to behold. In addition, from about mid-October through mid-May, the forest trails are mostly deserted, so solitude is another bonus. Finally,

Overleaf and opposite: *Rays of light through fog in Quinault Rain Forest (Trail 10)*

the wildlife comes down from the high country in the off-season, so you stand a very good chance of seeing animals, especially herds of elk, amid the greenery.

Governing Agencies

Most of the hikes in the western region are administered either by Olympic National Park or the Pacific Ranger District (Quinault Office) of the Olympic National Forest. A short section along the first part of the South Fork Hoh River Trail (Trail 9) is on Washington State Forest land under the jurisdiction of the Washington Department of Natural Resources.

TRAIL FEATURES TABLE

West Region: The Rain Forests

TRAIL	DIFFICULTY	LENGTH	TYPE	USES & ACCESS	TERRAIN	FLORA & FAUNA	OTHER
8	1	2.2	↻	👟 👫		🌲 🐦	👁
9	2	4.7	↗	👟 🎒 👫		🌲 🐦 🦌	👁
10	2	4.0	↻	👟 🐕 👫	🌊 🏞	🌲 🐦	
11	3–5	5.0–38.4	↗	👟 🎒 🐎	👣 🌊 🏞	🌲 🌸 🦌	👁 ⚒ 🏠
12	5	8.2	↗	👟 🎒 🐎 🐕	⛰ 👣	🌲	👁

USES & ACCESS	TYPE	TERRAIN	FLORA & FAUNA	OTHER
👟 Day Hiking	↻ Loop	⛰ Summit	🌲 Old-Growth Forest	👁 Viewpoint
🎒 Backpacking	↷ Semi-loop	👣 Steep	🌸 Wildflowers	⚒ Geologic Interest
🚵 Mountain Biking	↗ Out-and-back	🌊 Lake	🐦 Birds	🏠 Historic Interest
🐎 Horses		🏞 Waterfall	🦌 Wildlife	
🐕 Dogs Allowed	DIFFICULTY	🐟 Tidepool		
👫 Child-Friendly	- 1 2 3 4 5 + less more			

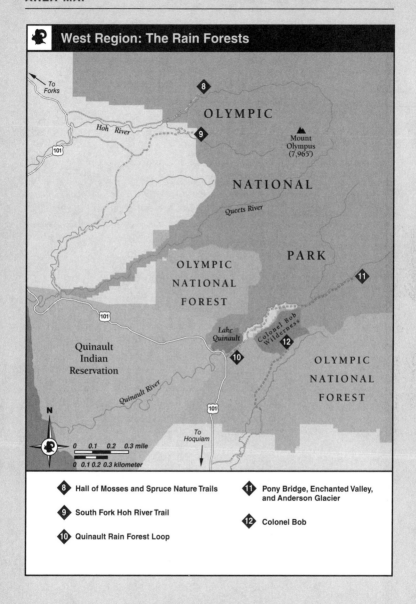

West Region: The Rain Forests

8 Hall of Mosses and Spruce Nature Trails

9 South Fork Hoh River Trail

10 Quinault Rain Forest Loop

11 Pony Bridge, Enchanted Valley, and Anderson Glacier

12 Colonel Bob

West Region: The Rain Forests

TRAIL 8

Day hiking,
child-friendly

2.2 miles

Loops

Difficulty: **1** 2 3 4 5

Hall of Mosses and Spruce Nature Trails 84

One of the most famous attractions in Olympic National Park—its amazingly dense and intensely green rain forests—is on spectacular display on these two easy and adjacent nature trails. You won't have these very popular trails to yourself, but that won't stop you from admiring the enormity of the trees, the delicacy of the ferns, and more shades of green than Crayola ever dreamed possible. This is the classic quick fix for a rain forest experience.

TRAIL 9

Day hiking, backpacking, child-friendly

4.7 miles

Out-and-back

Difficulty: 1 **2** 3 4 5

South Fork Hoh River Trail 90

A quiet alternative to the crowded trails in the famous Hoh Rain Forest, the South Fork Hoh River Trail is an off-the-beaten-path gem. Here, you'll enjoy all the same dense greenery, draping club mosses, and towering trees found in that busier destination, but you will likely enjoy more seclusion here. On the other hand, you will probably also have to deal with a muddy trail and a rough and confusing access road. But all good things come with a price, and here it is a more than reasonable price to pay.

TRAIL 10

Day hiking, dogs allowed, child-friendly

4.0 miles

Loop

Difficulty: 1 **2** 3 4 5

Quinault Rain Forest Loop 96

This is a conveniently located forest hike that offers more than just impressive trees for you to admire. Here you'll also discover fern-lined canyons, fine views of huge Lake Quinault, and a couple of small but attractive waterfalls. None of these features are outstanding, at least not when compared to some other hikes in this book, but taken together they make this relatively easy loop a real winner.

Pony Bridge, Enchanted Valley, and Anderson Glacier

There are options for everyone here on one of the best long trails in Olympic National Park. Day hikers can savor the deep forest on the lovely walk to Pony Bridge, where a scenic wooden bridge spans a dark, fern-lined canyon. Backpackers won't want to miss the trip to fittingly named Enchanted Valley with its abundant wildlife, waterfalls, and terrific views up to tall peaks. Hardy adventurers will delight in the even longer trip to the alpine country and spectacular viewpoint beside Anderson Glacier. No matter how far you go or how much time and energy you have, it's all outstanding.

TRAIL 11

Day hiking, backpacking, horses

5.0, 26.8, or 38.4 miles

Out-and-back

Difficulty: 1 2 **3** 4 **5**

Colonel Bob

A stiff climb leads to the best trail-accessible viewpoint in the western Olympics, with expansive vistas that stretch west to the vast Pacific Ocean, down to shimmering Lake Quinault, and north to the snowy landmark of Mount Olympus. It's not an easy viewpoint to reach, but it is definitely worth the effort.

TRAIL 12

Day hiking, backpacking, horses, dogs allowed

8.2 miles

Out-and-back

Difficulty: 1 2 3 4 **5**

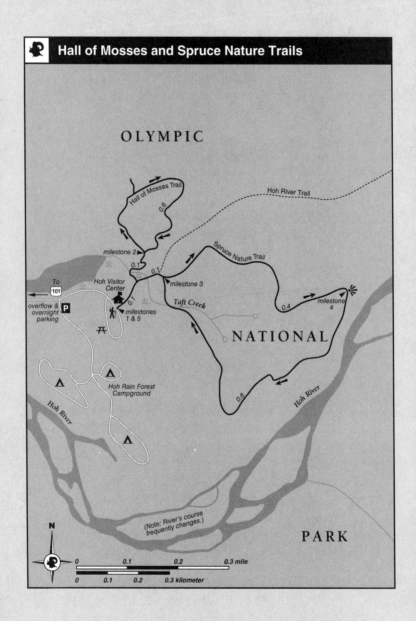

Hall of Mosses and Spruce Nature Trails

OLYMPIC

Hall of Mosses Trail

0.6

Hoh River Trail

milestone 2

0.1

Spruce Nature Trail

0.1

Hoh Visitor Center

To 101

milestone 3

0.1

overflow & overnight parking

P

Taft Creek

milestones 1 & 5

0.4

milestone 4

NATIONAL

Hoh Rain Forest Campground

0.6

Hoh River

Hoh River

(Note: River's course frequently changes.)

PARK

N

0   0.1   0.2   0.3 mile

0   0.1   0.2   0.3 kilometer

Hall of Mosses and Spruce Nature Trails

Perhaps the most renowned natural attraction of Olympic National Park is its temperate rain forests. Watered by prodigious amounts of rain, giant (make that massive, no, positively *enormous*) conifers tower up to 300 feet over the forest floor, creating a nearly unbroken canopy of branches and needles. Living exclusively in that high canopy are a host of unusual organisms, such as lettuce lichens, various mosses, and numerous small animals that spend their entire lives in the treetops and are rarely even seen by most people. At a lower level, shorter (but still quite large) trees, such as big-leaf maples, vine maples, and red alders, fill the available space and are literally covered with club mosses that drape off the branches like thick green hair that is up to 6 feet long. Shrubs, such as salmonberry, crowd into what niches they can find, while numerous ferns, liverworts, mosses, oxalis, and dozens of other plants carpet what is left of the uncovered forest floor. Green is literally everywhere, and it truly is a sight to behold.

There is no better place (and certainly no more famous place) to observe this unique ecosystem than in the Hoh Rain Forest, an easily accessible wonderland of green. The superbly named Hall of Mosses Trail hosts thousands of pedestrians—on summer weekends it often seems as though there are that many on a single day—looking for a quick fix rain forest experience. For a bit more exercise, you can include a second loop trip on the adjacent but somewhat less crowded Spruce Nature Trail, where the rain forest is a little less impressive, but which offers nice views of the Hoh River along the way.

TRAIL USE
Day hiking, child-friendly

LENGTH
2.2 miles (for both trails), 1–2 hours

CUMULATIVE ELEVATION
150'

DIFFICULTY
- **1** 2 3 4 5 +

TRAIL TYPE
Loops

SURFACE TYPE
Gravel

CONTOUR MAP
Trailhead brochures are sufficient.

START & END
N47° 51.618'
W123° 56.068'

FEATURES
Dense and drippy rain forest, moss-draped trees, large river

FACILITIES
Restrooms, picnic area, water, visitor center

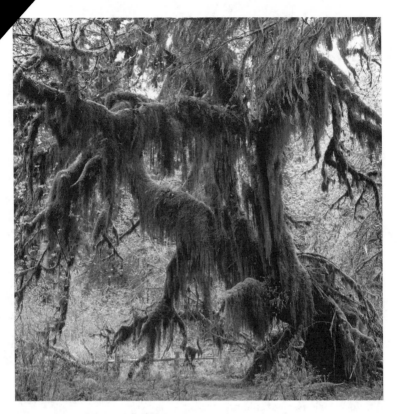

Moss-draped maple *in Hall of Mosses*

Best Time

The trails are open all year, though usually once or twice a winter, low-elevation snow and ice will temporarily close the access road. To avoid crowds, try to visit on a weekday in the shoulder seasons. A rainy day is a great time to visit because, well, this is a *rain* forest after all, and the moisture helps to bring out the vibrancy of the greens. In addition, rain tends to keep the casual tourists indoors, so the trail is less busy. For photographers, cloudy weather is actually preferred to avoid lighting contrast problems (but then, cloudy days far outnumber sunny ones anyway).

Finding the Trail

Drive US 101 about 11 miles south of Forks to the well-signed junction with Upper Hoh Road near milepost 178.4. Turn left (east), following signs to Hoh Rain Forest, and drive 13 miles to the park entrance station. Continue another 5.6 miles, watching carefully for elk in the surrounding forest as you drive, to the parking lot near the Hoh Visitor Center. Though the parking lot is quite large, on nice summer days it is often full, so you may be forced to leave your car in the overflow parking lot. This signed lot is located just off the campground access road about 0.2 mile west of the visitor center.

Trail Description

The level, gravel path starts a little south of the ranger station/visitor center ▶1 and goes northeast past a marshy area with some huge downed logs that have fallen into the muddy goo. Ferns and water-loving shrubs fill every nook and cranny of the forest floor. After only 120 yards, you come to a junction. The Hoh River Trail, which provides access to the Spruce Nature Trail and also serves as a long-distance hiking and backpacking route, goes straight, but you turn left on the Hall of Mosses Trail. Numerous interpretive signs along this route tell the story of this magical place—how different plants fill different ecological niches and how herds of elk create paths and keep the forest open by foraging—but while a little extra knowledge is always welcome, it's really the fun of gawking at all the big trees and dense greenery that makes this short hike so interesting.

 Old-Growth Forest

The trail crosses a bridge over a marshy section of spring-fed Taft Creek and then climbs a bit up a hillside to a fork at the start of the loop. ▶2 Turn left and walk by downed logs and enormous Sitka spruces, Douglas-firs, and western red cedars, some

Old-Growth Forest

of which are 300 feet tall. After a little more than 0.2 mile along this meandering loop, a short dead-end side trail goes left to a grove of big-leaf maples with abundant club mosses that hang up to 6 feet off their limbs. After almost 0.7 mile, the loop closes and you return back over the marsh to the junction with the Hoh River Trail.

If you have seen enough, you can turn right here and soon return to the trailhead. For a bit more exercise, however, why not include the rewarding loop walk on the nearby 1.2-mile Spruce Nature Trail? To find it, turn left (east) to cross a bridge over Taft Creek, and just 140 yards from the Hall of Mosses turnoff, reach the junction with the Spruce Nature Trail. ▶3 Turn right (southeast), walk 30 yards, and then come to the start of the loop. Turn left and begin your exploration of this lush river bottomland, where Douglas-firs, big-leaf maples, western hemlocks, and red alders grow to incredible sizes, and a wealth of small shrubs, ferns, mosses, herbs, liverworts, wildflowers, and grasses ensures that the lower levels of the forest are just as green as the upper ones. At the far end of this gentle loop is a nice little log bench beside the Hoh River. ▶4

Viewpoint

On one of those rare clear days, you will have nice views up the wide, gravel-strewn riverbed to several snowy peaks to the east. The river constantly changes course as floods and spring runoff move the channel around in the riverbed. In fact, only a few decades ago, the land you just walked through was part of the riverbed. While resting here, watch

Birds

for common mergansers, ospreys, bald eagles, and belted kingfishers, all of which call this river home.

The winding but nearly level trail follows the Hoh River downstream for almost 0.2 mile, passing many water-loving red alder trees that are used by bull elk to rub the velvet off their antlers in late summer. The trail then goes ever so slightly uphill to a small terrace that is above the more recent river channels. On this firmer ground, the conifers dominate and once again grow to prodigious sizes. At the close of the loop, you turn left and make the short walk back to the trailhead ▶5 the way you came.

Note: For a more satisfying exploration of this magnificent rain forest, consider a longer day hike or even a multiday backpacking trip on the Hoh River Trail, which begins at the same trailhead. This deservedly popular trail climbs very gradually on river-level bottomlands carpeted with greenery and towered over by humongous conifers. After 13 miles in this lush ecosystem, the trail leaves the river and climbs another 5 miles to the scenic alpine country around wildflower-filled Glacier Meadows and the rocky moraine at the foot of enormous Blue Glacier. The trail is a wonderful sampling of Olympic National Park, but it requires at least four days out of your vacation time to fully appreciate. In addition, you may need to reserve an overnight permit if you are camping at Elk Lake or Glacier Meadows on the upper parts of this trail. Day hikers can sample the best of the lowland forests by turning around at Happy Four Shelter after 5.8 miles.

🚶 MILESTONES

▶1	0.0	Visitor center parking lot (N47° 51.618' W123° 56.068')
▶2	0.2	Start of loop portion of the Hall of Mosses Trail (N47° 51.718' W123° 56.012')
▶3	1.0	Start of Spruce Nature Trail (N47° 51.676' W123° 55.992')
▶4	1.4	Bench beside Hoh River (N47° 51.650' W123° 55.478')
▶5	2.2	Return to parking lot (N47° 51.618' W123° 56.068')

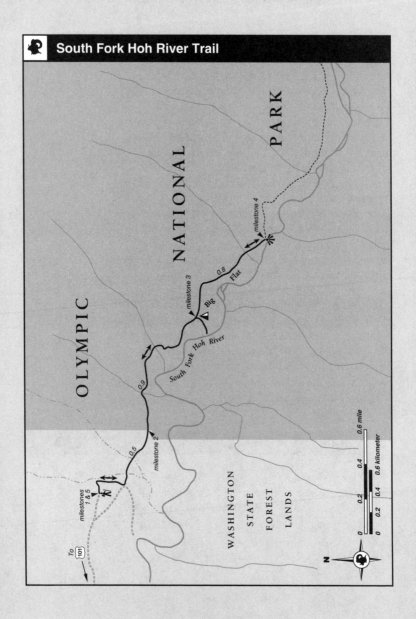

OLYMPIC

NATIONAL

PARK

milestone 4

0.8

Flat

milestone 3

Big

South Fork Hoh River

0.9

0.5

milestone 2

milestones 1 & 5

N

To 101

WASHINGTON
STATE
FOREST
LANDS

N

0   0.2   0.4   0.6 mile

0   0.2   0.4   0.6 kilometer

South Fork Hoh River Trail

So, you want to explore the rain forest but don't relish the thought of fighting the crowds of tourists in the Hoh. Well, have I got a secret for you. The nearby South Fork Hoh River goes through a rain forest valley that is nearly as grand as the larger main stem of the river, but it sees less than 1% of the visitors.

Of course, there are reasons for the lack of crowds. Chief among them is that the access road is unpaved and has plenty of potholes, and without good driving directions (see below), it's easy to get lost. In addition, unlike the nature paths in the Hoh Rain Forest, the trail here is not improved with gravel and, as a result, can be muddy. But if you don't care about those inconveniences, then this is the place for you. Just for fun, bring along a paint chart with every shade of green that the store sells, and then compare with Mother Nature to see how many the human manufacturers missed.

Best Time

The trail is usually open all year, though a few times each winter, low-elevation snow and ice will temporarily close the access road. Mud can be a problem, so the trail is better in the drier weather of summer or fall. This is a good hike for cloudy or drizzly days.

Finding the Trail

Note: It's easy to get lost on this drive, so please pay careful attention to your odometer and the driving directions on the following page.

TRAIL USE
Day hiking, backpacking, child-friendly

LENGTH
4.7 miles, 2.5 hours (including 0.3-mile side trip to the river from the Big Flat Campsite)

CUMULATIVE ELEVATION
350'

DIFFICULTY
- 1 **2** 3 4 5 +

TRAIL TYPE
Out-and-back

SURFACE TYPE
Dirt, mud

CONTOUR MAP
Green Trails *Mt Tom* #133 or Custom Correct *Mount Olympus Climber's Map*

START & END
N47° 47.972'
W123° 57.261'

FEATURES
Dense rain forest, solitude, beautiful river, wildlife

FACILITIES
None

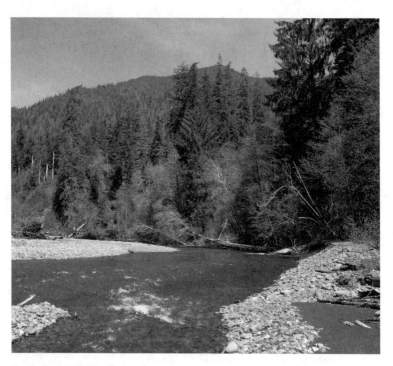

South Fork Hoh River *at Big Flat*

Drive US 101 about 13.5 miles south of Forks to milepost 176 and a well-signed junction with Clearwater Road. Turn left (east), following signs to Olympic Corrections Center, and go 7.1 miles to a junction with one-lane paved South Fork Hoh Road. Turn left, now following signs to South Hoh Campground; proceed 2.4 miles, and then veer right onto Maple Creek Road. The pavement ends 0.3 mile later, after which there are numerous (mostly small) potholes, though the road is still fine for passenger cars.

Exactly 5 miles after the end of pavement, you go left at an unsigned fork (staying on the main road) and 0.2 mile later cross a bridge over South Fork Hoh River. Less than 0.1 mile after the bridge is the turnoff to South Hoh Campground, which is on your right. Keep straight and drive 0.5 mile to an unsigned fork, where you go straight. Drive 1.8

miles and then go right at another unsigned fork. After 0.3 mile, you go straight where a road angles downhill to the right and reach the small road-end turnaround and trailhead in another 0.1 mile.

Trail Description

Starting in a dense moss-covered forest of relatively young Sitka spruces and western hemlocks, the needle-covered path descends from the parking area, ▶1 losing about 100 feet of elevation in just under 0.2 mile to a nearby gravel road. After almost touching this road at a curve in that vehicle route, your trail leaves civilization and enters a shady realm of intensely green second-growth forest. Sword ferns and mosses cover most of the rocky forest floor, while in May the blossoms of oxalis and trillium add white highlights to this land of green. Meanwhile, pioneer violets add appeal with their small but startlingly yellow blossoms. On sunny days (and, yes, they do happen on occasion), tiny pockets of dappled sunshine make it through the canopy to offer short periods of life-giving light to the plants below.

The trail soon crosses a normally dry creek bed, and then at 0.5 mile comes to the boundary of Olympic National Park ▶2 and a trail register. At this point, the trail leaves the second-growth forest and leads you into truly ancient and primeval woods. Several monstrous old trees and lots of gnarly stumps and downed logs provide plenty to admire in this old-growth forest. The up-and-down trail rarely gains or loses any significant elevation for the next 0.7 mile, so most of the walking is easy, if often rather muddy. For scenic variety, several small and seasonal creeks cross the trail as they tumble around moss-covered boulders. After nearly 1 mile, you cross a somewhat larger creek, where you may be forced to get your feet wet, especially after a heavy rain.

 Old-Growth Forest

At 1.4 miles, just after the trail completes a 100-foot descent, you come to a nice campsite. ▶3 This site is located in the middle of a large, relatively level area that goes by the descriptive (but rather unimaginative) name of Big Flat. Big-leaf maples, Sitka spruces, and western hemlocks, all festooned with hanging club mosses, provide visual appeal to this excellent lunch or overnight location. While here, don't miss the unsigned but obvious 0.15-mile side trail that goes to the right (south) from the camp to a gravel bar on the lovely South Fork Hoh River. If you are as lucky as I was, a leisurely rest stop by the river here may reward you with sightings of common mergansers, bald eagles, and river otters. This spot makes an excellent turnaround location for an easy hike.

Birds 🐦

Wildlife 🦌

If you are looking for more exercise, continue on the South Fork Hoh River Trail, which remains virtually level as it passes some particularly massive spruce trees right beside the trail. These giant conifers are perfectly designed to illicit awe in passing hikers. At 2.5 miles (including the 0.3-mile side trip from Big Flat Campsite), you come to the river again next to a large gravel bar. ▶4 Under clear skies, this forest opening offers pleasant views of the river and the nearby, heavily forested ridges. This peaceful location makes a good lunch spot and final turnaround point. For adventurous types, the official trail continues for another mile or so before ending at a large washout. Really adventurous and experienced hikers can skirt the washout and continue on an unmaintained and overgrown climber's route. That "trail," however, is too rugged to be recommended to rational hikers, most of whom have the sense to turn around at the gravel bar and return to the trailhead. ▶5

Viewpoint 📷

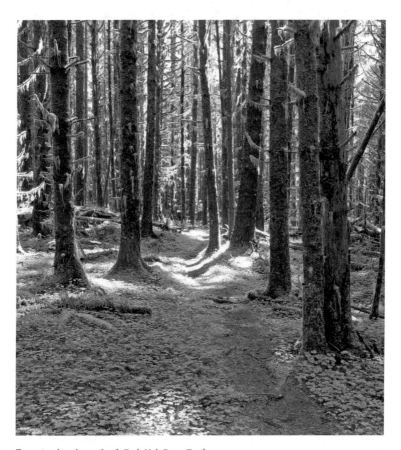

Forests *along lower South Fork Hoh River Trail*

🚶	**MILESTONES**		
►1	0.0	Take trail from parking area (N47° 47.972' W123° 57.261')	
►2	0.5	Enter Olympic National Park (N47° 47.717' W123° 56.769')	
►3	1.4	Big Flat Campsite (N47° 47.464' W123° 55.965')	
►4	2.5	Gravel bar on South Fork Hoh River (N47° 47.101' W123° 55.405')	
►5	4.7	Return to trailhead (N47° 47.972' W123° 57.261')	

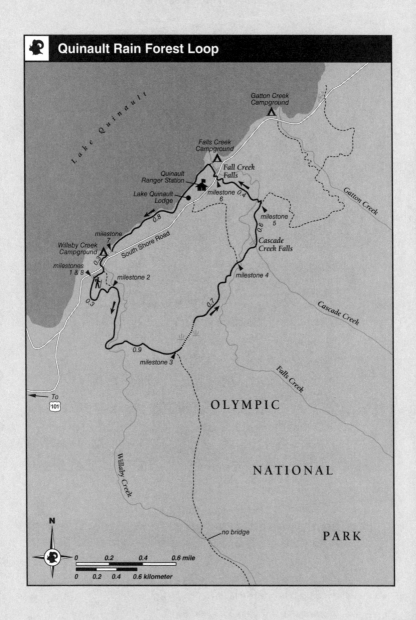

Quinault Rain Forest Loop

Quinault Rain Forest Loop

Conveniently located near Lake Quinault Lodge and three busy US Forest Service campgrounds, the trails in the Quinault Rain Forest are heavily used, but they remain well worth hiking, despite the crowds. Here you will discover impressive forests in all stages of development, from smaller second-growth trees to massive old-growth giants. The area also includes a couple of attractive fern-lined canyons, two small waterfalls, and lovely shoreline views of one of the largest lakes on the Olympic Peninsula. And all of this can be found along a fun 4-mile loop that can be completed in half a day and is located just a short distance off US 101. Ah, life is good for the hiker around here!

Best Time

The trail is usually open all year. A cloudy or even a rainy day is great for this forest walk, though for the best views of Lake Quinault, clear skies would be preferable.

Finding the Trail

Drive US 101 about 38 miles north of Hoquiam, and then turn right near milepost 125.6 onto South Shore Road. Proceed 1.2 miles on this good paved road and then turn right at a sign for the Rain Forest Nature Trail. Park in the large lot here.

TRAIL USE
Day hiking, dogs allowed, child-friendly

LENGTH
4.0 miles, 2 hours

CUMULATIVE ELEVATION
310'

DIFFICULTY
- 1 **2** 3 4 5 +

TRAIL TYPE
Loop

SURFACE TYPE
Dirt, gravel, boardwalk

CONTOUR MAP
Green Trails *Quinalt Lake* #197

START & END
N47° 27.580'
W123° 51.736'

FEATURES
Dense rain forest, small waterfalls, easily accessible trail, large lake

FACILITIES
Restrooms, picnic tables, trash can

Trail Description

The trail starts next to a large signboard at the east end of the parking area ▶1 across from the restrooms. After just a few yards, you reach a fork at the start of the Rain Forest Nature Trail loop. Either direction works, but it's a little more interesting to turn right, passing big moss-covered trees, downed nurse logs, and several interpretive signs with information about the rain forest ecosystem. The path winds its way uphill through this lush environment for 0.3 mile to a small kiosk and a junction. ▶2

Old-Growth Forest 🌳

The nature trail goes left, but for a more thorough sampling of this impressive forest, turn right on the Quinault Loop Trail. This path goes up and down past more big trees, some standing and others wind-toppled, to an overlook of a fern-lined gorge and a bridged crossing of Willaby Creek. Though the forest here is wet and drippy (it is a *rain* forest, after all), the mostly gravel trail is generally in good shape and not too muddy.

The trail now goes through a younger, second-growth forest and comes to a junction ▶3 at 1.2 miles. The trail to the right climbs almost 1,000 feet in 1.7 miles to its end at a huge, old Douglas-fir. The path is worth hiking, but there is no bridge at the crossing of Willaby Creek at the 1.1-mile point. Therefore, unless your trip is in the lower water season of midsummer to early fall, when you can reasonably ford the creek, it is better to skip this side trip.

The main trail goes left at the junction and soon crosses a long boardwalk over a large boggy area with lots of grasses, skunk cabbage, and scrubby cedar trees. From here, you reenter older forest and make your way along an easy but viewless trail to a junction ▶4 at 1.9 miles. The trail to the left is a shortcut route that descends to South Shore Road at Lake Quinault Lodge.

For the recommended loop, go right at the junction, cross a bridge over cascading Falls Creek,

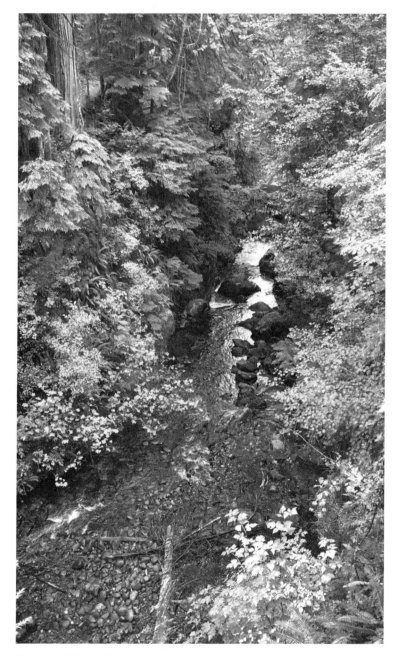

Gorge *on Willaby Creek*

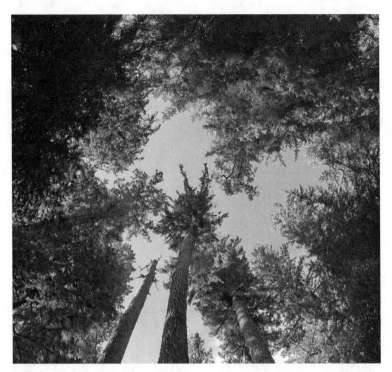

Looking skyward *amid tall trees in Quinault Rain Forest*

Waterfall 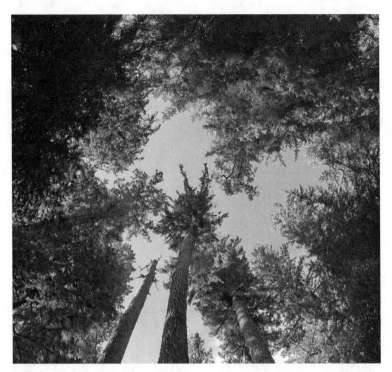 and soon come to smaller Cascade Creek that you cross just above sliding Cascade Creek Falls. Shortly after this is yet another junction. ▶5

You go left this time and make a couple of quick downhill switchbacks to a bridge over Falls Creek. The trail then winds downhill to the South Shore Road ▶6 and a secondary trailhead.

The recommended loop trail crosses the road and descends briefly to a fence enclosing a developed area with a manicured lawn and several **Waterfall** buildings. After following the outside of this fence for a short distance, you come to Falls Creek and a view of short Falls Creek Falls. The trail then turns downstream and takes you through a narrow 100-yard strip of forest between the creek on your right and a continuation of the fence on your left to a junction. The trail to the right crosses a bridge and leads to Falls Creek Campground.

You go left at this junction and for the next 0.6 mile follow the shoreline of large and beautiful Lake Quinault on a strip of forested land, with the lake on your right and the road and developed areas on your left. Look for bald eagles flying over the lake throughout the year and trumpeter swans resting on the water in the winter. You soon reach the lawn and buildings around quaint Lake Quinault Lodge. Walk past the lodge's small dock and then pass numerous lake viewpoints as the trail travels beneath a series of rustic private homes before coming to a junction with the access road into Willaby Creek Campground. ▶7

Go straight, walking along the road through the campground, until you reach the resumption of trail just past the restrooms near campsite 14. Go left on the trail, cross a concrete bridge over Willaby Creek, and then travel under the highway beneath that thoroughfare's bridge over the same stream. Just above this point is a junction with the Rain Forest Nature Trail. Go right, pass a truly monstrous Douglas-fir that is several hundred years old, and finish your hike with a short stroll back to the parking lot. ▶8

 Lake

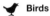 Birds

 Old-Growth Forest

🚶	**MILESTONES**	

▶1	0.0	Take trail from parking area (N47° 27.580' W123° 51.736')
▶2	0.3	Junction with nature trail loop (N47° 27.536' W123° 51.579')
▶3	1.2	Willaby Creek junction (N47° 27.264' W123° 51.035')
▶4	1.9	Junction with Lake Quinault Lodge trail (N47° 27.667' W123° 50.601')
▶5	2.5	Cascade Creek junction (N47° 27.920' W123° 50.455')
▶6	2.9	Cross South Shore Road (N47° 28.100' W123° 50.746')
▶7	3.7	Willaby Creek Campground road (N47° 27.763' W123° 51.534')
▶8	4.0	Return to trailhead (N47° 27.580' W123° 51.736')

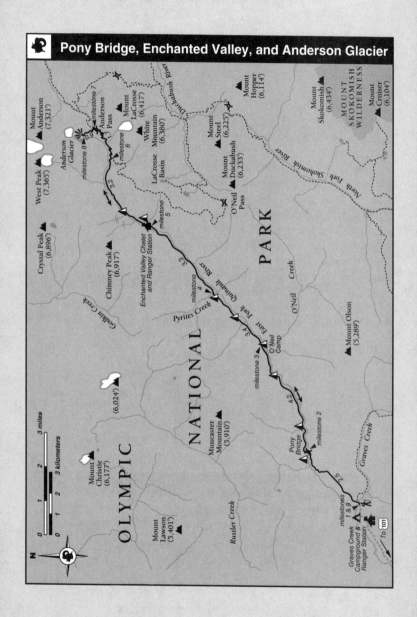

Pony Bridge, Enchanted Valley, and Anderson Glacier

Pony Bridge, Enchanted Valley, and Anderson Glacier

The East Fork Quinault River Trail is a long and outstandingly beautiful path that offers a wide variety of options, all of them superb, depending on your energy level, when you are visiting, and the amount of time you have available. If your time is limited, the hike to Pony Bridge is great fun in any season. The low-elevation rain forest is terrific, the wildlife (especially elk in the winter) is abundant, and the destination is a bridge spanning an extremely photogenic fern-lined canyon where a beautiful, clear river charges through a narrow chasm.

If you are up for a two- or three-day backpacking trip, there may be no better destination in the Olympics than wonderfully named Enchanted Valley. Renowned for its waterfalls and neck-craning mountain views, this deep valley is a delightful place to spend a night in the backcountry. Conveniently, Enchanted Valley is at its best in the spring, giving you a shoulder season option when other trails in the Olympic Mountains are still buried under several feet of snow. You even have an excellent chance of seeing wildlife, especially bears, so be sure to secure your food carefully.

For adventurous types with plenty of time and energy who are visiting in mid- to late summer, continuing the hike beyond Enchanted Valley to the icy grandeur of Anderson Glacier is a definite mustdo trip. This route takes you to one of the supreme high-elevation viewpoints in the range. Lots of ice, wildflowers, and mountain views make this a spot that every backpacker in the Olympic Mountains simply must see at least once in his or her hiking life. If you want to see the actual glacier, however, you better hurry because it is now practically gone.

TRAIL USE
Day hiking, backpacking, horses (but rare)

LENGTH
Bridge: 5.0 miles, 2.5–3 hours; Valley: 26.8 miles, 2–4 days; Glacier: 38.4 miles, 3–5 days

CUMULATIVE ELEVATION
960' to Bridge; 2,450' to Valley; 5,750' to Glacier

DIFFICULTY
- 1 2 **3 4 5** +

TRAIL TYPE
Out-and-back

SURFACE TYPE
Dirt, gravel

CONTOUR MAP
Custom Correct *Enchanted Valley–Skokomish* or Green Trails *Mt Christie* #166 and *Mt Steel* #167

START & END
N47° 34.365'
W123° 34.209'

FEATURES
Rain forest, river, wildlife, waterfalls, mountain views

FACILITIES
Restrooms, trash can

Best Time

The day hike to Pony Bridge is usually open all year, though a few times each winter, flooding or low-elevation snow and ice will temporarily close the access road. This portion of the hike is good for a cloudy or rainy day. For solitude and wildlife (especially elk), winter is ideal. Mud can be a problem in the winter, however, so wear boots rather than tennis shoes.

The trail as far as Enchanted Valley is usually hikable late April–November. It is great throughout the hiking season, but mid- to late May is probably the most spectacular time because the waterfalls will be at their most impressive then. Fall (mid-October) is also beautiful.

The trail to Anderson Glacier is open from about late July to October. Early August is best for wildflowers, while September is great for picking huckleberries. Early to mid-October offers wonderful fall colors. Good weather is required to enjoy the views.

Finding the Trail

Drive US 101 about 38 miles north of Hoquiam, and then turn right near milepost 125.6 onto paved South Shore Road. After 2.2 miles, you drive past the Quinault Ranger Station, where backpackers

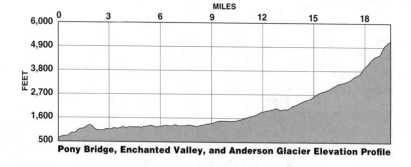

Pony Bridge, Enchanted Valley, and Anderson Glacier Elevation Profile

should stop to fill out a wilderness permit. The pavement ends after another 5.8 miles. Now on a good gravel road, you drive 4.2 miles to the boundary of Olympic National Park. Exactly 1 mile later (a total of 13.2 miles from US 101), you go straight at a junction, where the road going left immediately crosses a bridge over the Quinault River. Now on narrow Graves Creek Road, you slowly proceed a final 6.4 miles to the road-end trailhead, shortly after you pass the signed turnoff to Graves Creek Campground.

Trail Description

The trail begins from the northeast end of the parking area ▶1 and almost immediately crosses a high wooden bridge over Graves Creek. At 0.1 mile is a prominently signed junction. Keep straight on the trail to Enchanted Valley and for the next 1.8 miles follow a fairly wide, mostly gravel trail that is actually an overgrown old road. Elk are abundant here—one of the largest herds of elk in the world lives in the Quinault River drainage—especially in winter when most of the animals are down from the high country. Even without the wildlife, however, the surrounding area is a gloriously lush rain forest of moss-draped maples and towering firs, spruces, hemlocks, and cedars. Beneath the canopy is the usual dense understory of mixed greens to enjoy, including dozens of varieties of shrubs, mosses, ferns, mushrooms, grasses, and lichens.

 Wildlife

 Old-Growth Forest

You cross a small side creek on a log bridge, make a quick uphill, and then travel on the level or intermittently uphill path through the forest, constantly awed by the size of many of these ancient trees. At 1.9 miles, the trail narrows where the old road ends beside a decaying picnic table atop a little rise. From here, you lose about 200 feet in the next 0.6 mile to Pony Bridge. ▶2 This scenic wooden span over a narrow chasm carved by the remarkably clear East Fork Quinault River offers fine views of the shady, fern-lined gorge. The bridge makes an excellent day hike goal, but you could also spend the night here because there is a nice camp on your left just after the bridge crossing.

Hikers continuing beyond Pony Bridge soon begin a pattern that will remain true for the next 10 miles: lots of small ups and downs as the trail makes its way through dense rain forest on the hillside above the East Fork Quinault River. Along the way, there are a handful of small and inviting riverside camps and several opportunities to visit the river and enjoy its soothing charms. Much of the way is on river-level flats covered with ferns and moss-draped maples, and there are a number of pretty little side creeks for **Wildlife** variety. In September you will probably hear the odd high-pitched sounds of elk bugling and maybe even see some of the buglers as well. The trail is entirely viewless but great fun every step of the way. At 6.7 miles, you come to a junction with the signed side trail to O'Neil Camp. ▶3

The main trail goes straight at this junction and wanders through more fine forests for another 3.4 miles to Pyrites Creek Camp, which is located just before you cross—you guessed it—Pyrites Creek. ▶4 Near 12.9 miles, you pass through a curious wooden gate that seems to have no obvious discernible purpose (rangers say that the gate serves to hold in pack animals that occasionally come up here and escape from their handlers). You then **Historic Interest** cross a narrow log bridge over the river and soon come to the opening of Enchanted Valley and the historic three-story Enchanted Valley Chalet. ▶5 This attractive old three-story building was once open to guests but now serves as a seasonal ranger cabin. The designated backpacker's camping area is **Wildlife** located just beyond the chalet. *Warning:* Black bears are very common in and around Enchanted Valley. Be sure to properly store all food (and anything else that smells even remotely interesting) away from the bruins at all times.

Long, narrow, and relatively open, Enchanted Valley sits in an idyllic mountain setting. Dark and imposing cliffs and rocky ridges tower above the valley, leaving you with a sore neck just from taking in the scenery. The highest point, Chimney Peak, rises nearly 5,000 vertical feet almost directly from the valley floor. You can also see the tall snow-covered pinnacles of West Peak and Mount Anderson at the head of the valley. In late spring and early summer, hundreds of waterfalls streak down the cliffs that enclose the valley, giving this place its other common name: Valley of 1,000 Waterfalls.

 Viewpoint

 Waterfall

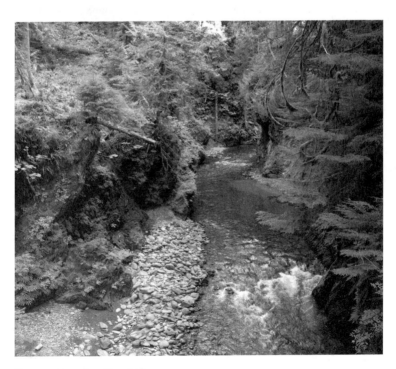

Gorge *upstream from Pony Bridge*

Enchanted Valley is certainly reward enough for your efforts, but for even more great scenery, make a base camp in the valley and take a day hike up to Anderson Glacier. To reach it, continue hiking on the main trail as it goes up and down for 0.8 mile to a good campsite in the upper part of Enchanted Valley. From there, it's mostly uphill in forest, with several crossings of small creeks along the way. As you climb, you'll catch enticing glimpses of the tall spire of West Peak to the north–northwest. You cross a loudly tumbling creek on a log bridge and then at 3.2 miles from the Enchanted Valley Chalet come to a boulder-strewn landslide and a junction. ►6 O'Neil Pass and the magnificent La Crosse Basin lie to the right—a wonderful extension of your backpacking trip if you have a couple of extra days.

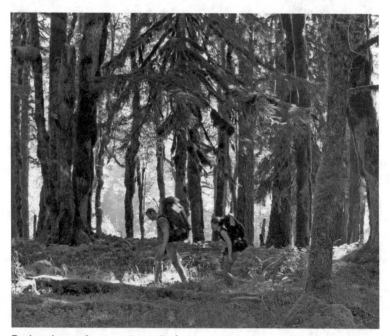

Backpackers *in forest near Pyrites Creek*

For the Anderson Glacier, keep straight at the junction and climb a series of switchbacks and traverses. The brushy slopes here are kept clear of trees by frequent avalanches. As a result, this relatively open terrain offers good views of Chimney Peak and Enchanted Valley and provides plenty of sunshine for an abundant huckleberry crop. The berries peak from late August to mid-September, which is also the ideal time to see black bears, which congregate here to feast on the fruit. After 10 switchbacks, you top out at a campsite, shallow pond, and trail junction at Anderson Pass. ▶7

Viewpoint

Wildlife

The view from the pass is nice but hardly overwhelming. For the truly grand scenery, you must turn left (uphill) at the junction, following signs to Anderson Glacier. This path climbs numerous short and often steep switchbacks on an open slope carpeted with heather, wildflowers, and, most notably, huckleberry bushes. In early September these bushes offer a treat for the taste buds with their delicious berries, while in mid-October they provide a treat for the eyes with acres of bright red leaves. At the top of the slope, you pass above a shallow lakelet, and then make a final rocky climb to the top of an old moraine and (finally) the promised superb viewpoint. ▶8

Steep

Wildflowers

Viewpoint

Directly in front of you is a large meltwater lake, usually filled with icebergs through the entire summer, and the snow-streaked jagged crags of towering Mount Anderson. Anderson Glacier sits in the bowl between the peak and the lake. Not so many years ago, this was one of the largest glaciers in the Olympic Mountains, filling this entire basin and covering most of the lake. Today, the ice field is a tiny fragment of its former self and will probably very soon cease to be a glacier at all. But the scenery will still be outstanding, so don't cancel a visit just because of a diminished glacier. Be sure to take the time to explore other viewpoints on the old moraine, from

Lake

Geologic
Interest

which you will be able to look down to Enchanted Valley and southeast, across Anderson Pass, to rugged Mount La Crosse and White Mountain. If you are feeling ambitious, you can even scramble down to the lake. Having enjoyed this dramatic spot for as long as time allows, turn around and make the long, scenic journey back to Enchanted Valley and the trailhead ▶9 the way you came.

🚶 MILESTONES

▶1	0.0	Take trail from parking area (N47° 34.365' W123° 34.209')
▶2	2.5	Pony Bridge (N47° 35.800' W123° 32.467')
▶3	6.7	Spur trail to O'Neil Camp (N47° 36.943' W123° 28.606')
▶4	10.1	Pyrites Creek (N47° 38.440' W123° 25.999')
▶5	13.4	Enchanted Valley Chalet (N47° 40.276' W123° 23.357')
▶6	16.6	O'Neil Pass junction (N47° 41.337' W123° 20.648')
▶7	18.3	Anderson Pass (N47° 41.768' W123° 19.591')
▶8	19.2	Anderson Glacier viewpoint (N47° 42.055' W123° 19.789')
▶9	38.4	Return to trailhead (N47° 34.365' W123° 34.209')

Colonel Bob

The summit of Colonel Bob is easily the best trail-accessible viewpoint in the western Olympics. That is not to say, however, that Colonel Bob is easily accessible by trail. It's a tough climb, but this just makes the rewards at trail's end that much more satisfying. And what rewards! Views from this high, rocky perch extend well out over the Pacific Ocean, down to the shimmering blue waters of Lake Quinault, and north to the icy mass of Mount Olympus. When you throw in additional vistas that include hundreds of rugged ridges and canyons in all directions, then you have a view that is well worth all that sweat.

Best Time

The trail is usually open late June–October. It is good any time that it's open, but you will definitely need a clear day to enjoy the sights.

Finding the Trail

Drive US 101 to a junction near milepost 112.6, about 25.5 miles north of Hoquiam. Turn east onto Donkey Creek Road (also known as Forest Road 22) and go 8.4 miles on this paved logging road to a major signed junction. You turn left (north) onto FR 2204, go 3.1 miles to the end of the pavement, and then proceed another 1.1 miles to a junction immediately after a tall bridge over the Humptulips River. Go right and drive a final 7.3 miles to the signed trailhead. Parking is on the right.

TRAIL USE
Day hiking, backpacking, horses, dogs allowed

LENGTH
8.2 miles, 4.5 hours or 2 days

CUMULATIVE ELEVATION
3,520'

DIFFICULTY
- 1 2 3 4 **5** +

TRAIL TYPE
Out-and-back

SURFACE TYPE
Dirt

CONTOUR MAP
Custom Correct *Quinault–Colonel Bob* or Green Trails *Grisdale* #198

START & END
N47° 27.427'
W123° 43.896'

FEATURES
High viewpoint, forests

FACILITIES
Restrooms

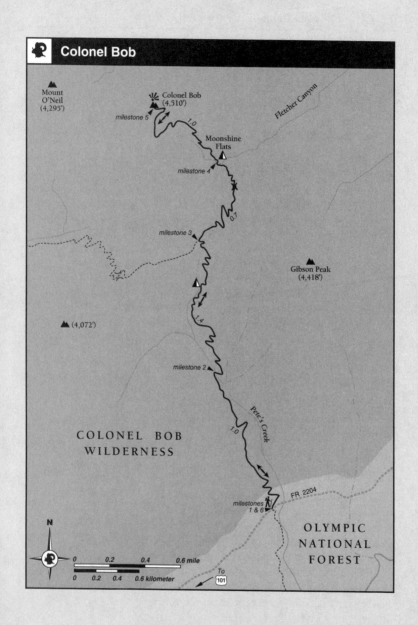

Colonel Bob

Mount O'Neil (4,295')

Colonel Bob (4,510')

milestone 5

1.0

Fletcher Canyon

Moonshine Flats

milestone 4

0.7

milestone 3

Gibson Peak (4,418')

▲ (4,072')

1.4

milestone 2

COLONEL BOB WILDERNESS

Pete's Creek

1.0

milestones 1 & 6

FR 2204

OLYMPIC NATIONAL FOREST

N

0   0.2   0.4   0.6 mile

0   0.2   0.4   0.6 kilometer

To 101

Trail Description

Take the upper portion of Pete's Creek Trail, which goes uphill directly across the road from the parking area. ▶1 This trail has a bit more than 3,500 feet of climbing to accomplish, and only about 4 miles in which to do it, so there's no sense in wasting time, a necessity that the trail builders clearly recognized as well. As a result, you immediately begin ascending, often steeply, on a hillside covered with a thick forest of western red cedars, Douglas-firs, and western hemlocks. As always in the western Olympics, the understory is a thick mass of green shrubs, ferns, mosses, lichens, and other plants in species beyond listing. The "river music" of tumbling Pete's Creek provides audio accompaniment to the visual scenery all around.

 Old-Growth Forest

After 1 mile of rounded switchbacks, you cross Pete's Creek ▶2 at a point where the water usually flows under the rocky creek bed. In 2012 there was a picturesque but precariously skinny 5-foot-tall rock cairn just downstream from this crossing.

More switchbacks (many more) interspersed with long uphill traverses (plenty of those too) now take you up the wooded slopes of Gibson Peak. You pass a nice campsite at 1.9 miles and less than 0.1 mile later begin zigzagging up a brushy avalanche slope. From here, you gain the first decent views of

 Viewpoint

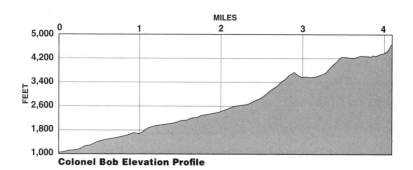

Colonel Bob Elevation Profile

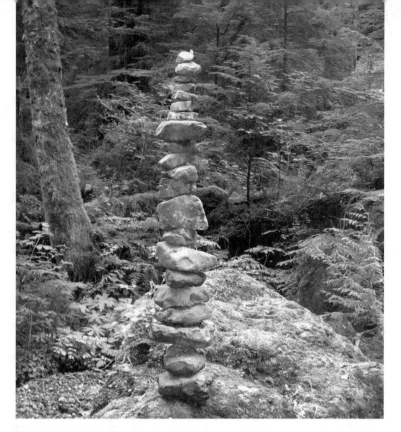

Tall cairn *at Pete's Creek*

Steep

the mostly forested craggy peaks that surround you. At 2.4 miles is a junction with Colonel Bob Trail. ▶3

You turn sharply right here (uphill, of course) and continue plodding up a series of often steep switchbacks. After climbing more of the fairly open avalanche chute, you reenter forest and top a low ridge beside a forested saddle. From here, you actually descend almost 100 feet (don't worry; you'll gain it all back), pass a good view down the steep defile of Fletcher Canyon, and then wander past tiny ponds, large boulders, and pretty heather meadows to a crossing of the trickling creek in Moonshine Flats. ▶4 There are nice camps in this area featuring good views up to the rocky summit of Colonel Bob, still about 1,000 feet above you.

More climbing, some of the steepest thus far, takes you to Colonel Bob's narrow summit ridge, where you turn right and head straight for the imposing rocky top of the peak. After a short up-and-down traverse, the final push is up steps carved in the rock. Upon reaching Colonel Bob's summit, ▶5 you finally get to appreciate the promised views. Nearby are numerous craggy peaks, but it's the more-distant vistas west to the vast Pacific Ocean and much smaller (but still respectably large) Lake Quinault; north to the glacier-clad glory of Mount Olympus; and east to the snowy dome of Mount Rainier that will grab most of your attention. Soak it all in, and then reluctantly bow to the pressures of time and head back to the trailhead ▶6 the way you came.

 Steep

 Summit

 Viewpoint

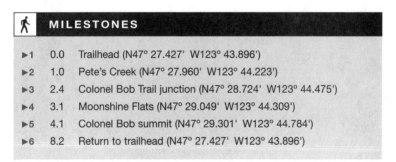

		MILESTONES
▶1	0.0	Trailhead (N47° 27.427' W123° 43.896')
▶2	1.0	Pete's Creek (N47° 27.960' W123° 44.223')
▶3	2.4	Colonel Bob Trail junction (N47° 28.724' W123° 44.475')
▶4	3.1	Moonshine Flats (N47° 29.049' W123° 44.309')
▶5	4.1	Colonel Bob summit (N47° 29.301' W123° 44.784')
▶6	8.2	Return to trailhead (N47° 27.427' W123° 43.896')

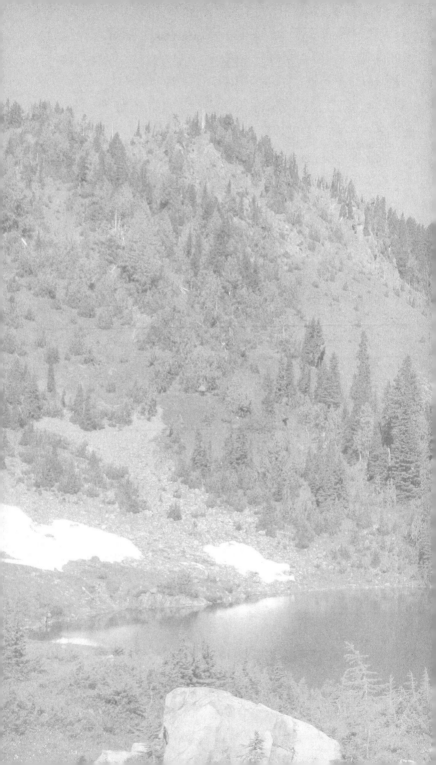

CHAPTER 3

Northwest Region: Lake Crescent and Sol Duc Areas

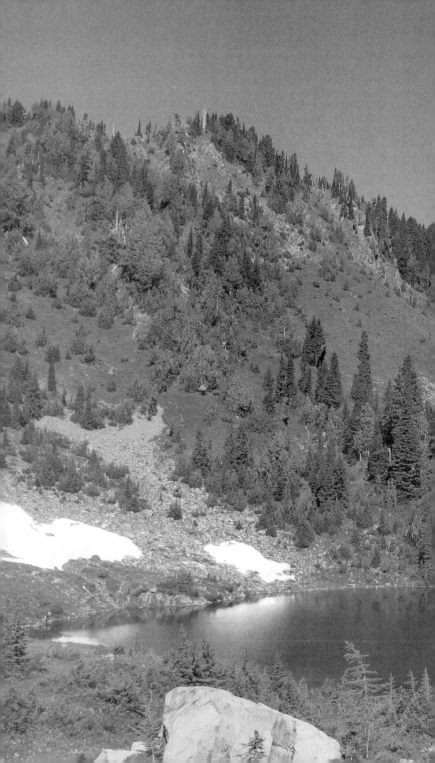

Northwest Region: Lake Crescent and Sol Duc Areas

Centered on two of Olympic National Park's finest attractions—huge and very scenic Lake Crescent and the deep, green valley of the Sol Duc River—the northwest region is one of the most popular hiking and camping areas on the Olympic Peninsula. The forests here are less lush than in the rain forests just a few miles to the southwest, but they are still mighty impressive and the lack of a "rain" forest necessarily means that the weather here is *relatively* drier and sunnier than in those soggy environs.

The general topography here is typical of the Olympic Peninsula, dense forests covering steep ridges and bisected by beautiful, clear streams. Those streams are sprinkled with waterfalls, which make great hiking destinations, while the ridges offer hikers delights in the form of wildflower-covered meadows and outstanding views. In some areas, wildlife is extremely common, in particular black bears along the High Divide, so keep your eyes open and guard your food carefully.

The Sol Duc Valley and its surrounding high country is, perhaps, the best all-around sampler of what the Olympic Mountains have to offer. It is a microcosm of the ecosystem with some of the best of all the area's main attractions. Here you'll find one of the peninsula's most beautiful rivers, on which is one of the region's most impressive waterfalls, all surrounded by some of the area's prettiest forests. And then, arguably even better, you have the surrounding high-elevation ridges. These alpine wonderlands, especially High Divide, offer perhaps the peninsula's most beautiful mountain lakes, some of its best on-trail views, incredibly impressive wildflower displays, and outstanding wildlife habitat. For hikers with only limited time, this is the place to explore. Of course, others agree with this assessment, so the trails are extremely popular and getting an overnight permit can be a challenge.

Overleaf and opposite: *Round Lake in Seven Lakes Basin (Trail 15)*

Long, very deep, and backed by tall ridges, enormous Lake Crescent has been described as looking like a freshwater fjord. The lake is also incredibly pure and clear, not to mention very scenic, so the list of attributes is impressive. Several trails explore this lake and its surrounding terrain, most of them short, and all of them very beautiful.

By Olympic standards, this region, especially Lake Crescent and along the Strait of Juan de Fuca, enjoys a fairly mild climate. The low-elevation trails near the lake and along the beaches are usually hikable all year, and there are noticeably fewer clouds and less rain here than just a short distance to the southwest. (This is not to imply that it is arid or anything—we're talking in relative terms here, folks.) The high country, on the other hand, gets enormous amounts of snow, and its aspect on the slopes, especially in the Seven Lakes Basin on the north side of High Divide, means that the white stuff takes an unusually long time to melt away. In some years, it never does, but most summers find enough of the snow gone by late July or early August to make the high trails hikable.

Governing Agencies

The Mount Muller Loop (Trail 13) is in the Olympic National Forest and is administered by the Pacific Ranger District (Forks Office). The hike to The Cove (Trail 19) is under the jurisdiction of Clallam County Parks and the Washington Department of Natural Resources. All other hikes in this region are in Olympic National Park.

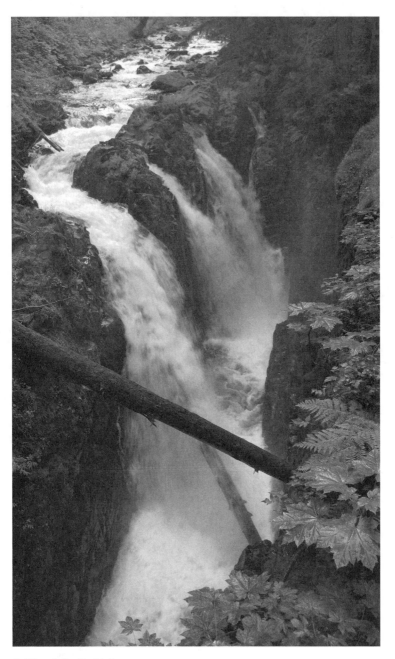

Sol Duc Falls *(Trail 14)*

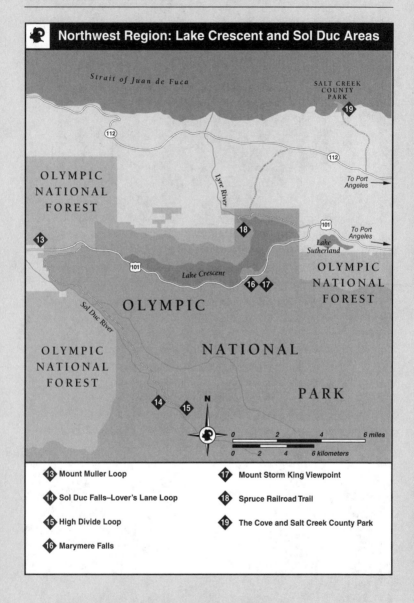

Northwest Region: Lake Crescent and Sol Duc Areas

Strait of Juan de Fuca

SALT CREEK
COUNTY
PARK

19

112

OLYMPIC
NATIONAL
FOREST

Lyre River

112

To Port
Angeles

18

13

101

To Port
Angeles

Lake
Sutherland

101

Lake Crescent

OLYMPIC
NATIONAL
FOREST

16 **17**

Sol Duc River

OLYMPIC

OLYMPIC
NATIONAL
FOREST

NATIONAL

14 **15**

N

PARK

| 0 | | 2 | | 4 | | 6 miles |

| 0 | 2 | 4 | 6 kilometers |

13 Mount Muller Loop

14 Sol Duc Falls–Lover's Lane Loop

15 High Divide Loop

16 Marymere Falls

17 Mount Storm King Viewpoint

18 Spruce Railroad Trail

19 The Cove and Salt Creek County Park

Northwest Region: Lake Crescent and Sol Duc Areas

TRAIL	DIFFICULTY	LENGTH	TYPE	USES & ACCESS	TERRAIN	FLORA & FAUNA	OTHER
13	5	13.0	Loop	Day Hiking, Mountain Biking, Horses, Dogs Allowed	Summit	Wildflowers, Birds	Viewpoint, Geologic Interest
14	2	5.9	Loop	Day Hiking, Child-Friendly	Waterfall	Old-Growth Forest, Wildflowers, Birds	Historic Interest
15	5	20.3	Loop	Backpacking, Horses	Summit, Steep, Lake, Waterfall	Old-Growth Forest, Wildflowers, Wildlife	Viewpoint
16	1	1.6	Out-and-back	Day Hiking, Child-Friendly	Lake, Waterfall	Old-Growth Forest	
17	3	3.2	Out-and-back	Day Hiking	Steep, Lake		Viewpoint
18	2	5.8	Out-and-back	Day Hiking, Mountain Biking, Horses, Dogs Allowed, Child-Friendly	Lake	Wildflowers	Viewpoint, Historic Interest
19	2	2.2	Out-and-back	Day Hiking, Dogs Allowed, Child-Friendly	Steep, Tidepool		Viewpoint

USES & ACCESS	TYPE	TERRAIN	FLORA & FAUNA	OTHER
Day Hiking	Loop	Summit	Old-Growth Forest	Viewpoint
Backpacking	Semi-loop	Steep	Wildflowers	Geologic Interest
Mountain Biking	Out-and-back	Lake	Birds	Historic Interest
Horses		Waterfall	Wildlife	
Dogs Allowed	DIFFICULTY	Tidepool		
Child-Friendly	- 1 2 3 4 5 + less more			

Northwest Region:
Lake Crescent and Sol Duc Areas

TRAIL 13

Day hiking, mountain biking, horses, dogs allowed

13.0 miles

Loop

Difficulty: 1 2 3 4 **5**

Mount Muller Loop 126

This relatively new trail is not yet on the radar screens of most hikers, but that is bound to change once word gets out about the ridgetop views and wildflower displays along this long and challenging loop. It's not an easy hike, but it's enjoyable.

TRAIL 14

Day hiking, child-friendly

5.9 miles

Loop

Difficulty: 1 **2** 3 4 5

Sol Duc Falls–Lover's Lane Loop . . . 133

Although thousands of people take the short and easy trail to beautiful Sol Duc Falls, few know about this longer woodsy loop to the same destination. But the extra distance is rewarded with fine forest and river scenery, a chance to visit a lesser-known nearby waterfall, and good exercise on a little-traveled trail. All of which allows you to commune with nature and really immerse yourself in the forest's many charms.

TRAIL 15

Backpacking, horses

20.3 miles

Loop

Difficulty: 1 2 3 4 **5**

High Divide Loop 140

Probably the premier on-trail backpacking trip in the Olympic Mountains, the High Divide Loop soon leaves authors struggling to find enough superlative adjectives. Here you will find some of the best views, alpine lakes, wildflower displays, and wildlife habitat of any place in the range. Not surprisingly, you will also find one of the largest populations of backpackers in the park. Don't expect solitude, and apply early for a reserved permit; once on the trail, simply revel in the glories.

Marymere Falls 152

This path is a perfect choice for car-bound tourists looking for a good but not too difficult leg stretcher. The destination is a beautiful little waterfall, but the trail also has fine forests to explore and good spots for kids to play along a forest stream. Visit on a weekday under cloudy (or even rainy) skies to avoid most of the crowds.

TRAIL 16

Day hiking,
child-friendly
1.6 miles
Out-and-back
Difficulty: **1** 2 3 4 5

Mount Storm King Viewpoint 156

Here is a short but steep trail that leads to a dizzying viewpoint on a rocky ridge high on the side of Mount Storm King. The views down to Lake Crescent and across to Pyramid Mountain are superb, and the stiff climb weeds out the casual hikers, so you may even have the view all to yourself.

TRAIL 17

Day hiking
3.2 miles
Out-and-back
Difficulty: 1 2 **3** 4 5

Spruce Railroad Trail 161

This is a nearly flat trail right along the shores of large and very scenic Lake Crescent that follows the course of a historic railroad line. The lake views are outstanding, the early summer wildflowers are a joy, and you even have a chance to see wildlife and check out an old railroad tunnel.

TRAIL 18

Day hiking, mountain
biking, horses, dogs
allowed, child-friendly
5.8 miles
Out-and-back
Difficulty: 1 **2** 3 4 5

The Cove and Salt Creek County Park 166

Salt Creek County Park, a little gem on the shores of the Strait of Juan de Fuca, is popular with locals but usually overlooked by visitors to the region. If you avoid that same mistake, you'll be treated to some of the peninsula's best tidepooling, dramatic coastal scenery, and an easy but uncrowded trail to a lovely little cove.

TRAIL 19

Day hiking, dogs
allowed, child-friendly
2.2 miles
Out-and-back
Difficulty: 1 **2** 3 4 5

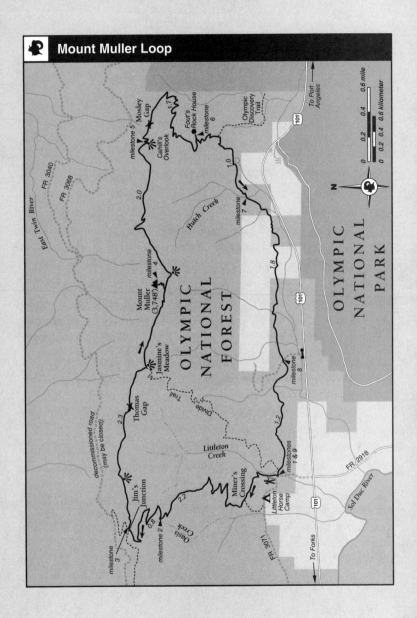

Mount Muller Loop

Mosley Gap

milestone 5

Cahill's Overlook

Fout's Rock House

milestone 6

Olympic Discovery Trail

.7

1.0

milestone 7

Hutch Creek

2.0

milestone 4

Mount Muller (3,748')

1.8

101

To Port Angeles

OLYMPIC NATIONAL PARK

FR 3040

FR 3068

East Twin River

Jasmine's Meadow

OLYMPIC NATIONAL FOREST

Divide Trail

Thomas Gap

2.3

decommissioned road (may be closed)

milestone 8

1.2

Littleton Creek

Jim's Junction

Miner's Crossing

milestones 1 & 9

FR 2918

Sol Duc River

milestone 3

milestone 2

0.8

2.2

Oasis Creek

Littleton Horse Camp

FR 3071

To Forks

101

N

0   0.2   0.4   0.6 kilometer

0   0.2   0.4   0.6 mile

Mount Muller Loop

Despite its many merits, the Mount Muller Loop is not heavily used, mostly because it is a relatively new trail and people have not yet become aware of its charms. That is bound to change, however, as hikers discover that this well-maintained route offers one of the finest ridge walks on the Olympic Peninsula. The trail also has seasonal wildflower displays, ridgetop meadows, and some of the best views in this part of the range. On the downside, the loop is quite long and involves a considerable elevation gain. But for strong hikers who aren't dissuaded by the physical challenge, this trip is hard to beat. *Note:* A brand-new cutoff trail offers a woodsy, switchbacking return route from Jasmine's Meadow back to the trailhead. This new trail offers an option for those looking to shorten this long hike.

Best Time

The trail is usually open mid-May–October and is good any time that it's open. The trip is especially appealing when the wildflowers are blooming in June and early July. A clear day is much better to enjoy the excellent views.

Finding the Trail

Drive US 101 to a junction near milepost 216.5 (about 24.5 miles north and east of Forks or 32 miles west of Port Angeles). Turn north onto Forest Road 3071, following signs to Mount Muller/ Littleton Loop Trailhead, and drive this narrow gravel road for 0.4 mile to the signed trailhead parking area on the right.

TRAIL USE
Day hiking, mountain biking, horses, dogs allowed

LENGTH
13.0 miles (including 0.2-mile side trip to the top of Mount Muller), 7 hours

CUMULATIVE ELEVATION
3,140'

DIFFICULTY
- 1 2 3 4 **5** +

TRAIL TYPE
Loop

SURFACE TYPE
Dirt

CONTOUR MAP
Custom Correct *Lake Crescent–Happy Lake Ridge*

START & END
N48° 04.552'
W124° 00.784'

FEATURES
Ridgetop viewpoints, wildflower-filled meadows, relative solitude

FACILITIES
Restrooms

Trail Description

Both ends of this loop depart directly from the parking lot. ▶1 For a clockwise loop (the preferred direction because it allows you to do most of the climbing in the beginning), you go left beside a large trailhead signboard and climb gradually through a young forest of Douglas-firs, western hemlocks, and red alders. In less than 0.1 mile, you come to seasonal Littleton Creek and follow this attractive forest-lined brook upstream. At just under 0.3 mile, the trail switchbacks to the left and climbs away from the creek. A second switchback comes 100 yards later, and then you begin an extended, moderately graded ascent that steadily takes you up a forested south-facing hillside.

At 0.6 mile, you cross a long-abandoned jeep track that a sign identifies as Miner's Crossing. Today, the uphill portion of the old jeep track is badly overgrown, but the downhill section serves as an equestrian connector trail to the Littleton Horse Camp.

Your trail continues straight and immediately resumes climbing, though eight moderately long switchbacks keep the grade from being steep. After the first series of switchbacks, a long northwesterly traverse leads to a second set of switchbacks. At the third in this series is a junction with a 15-yard side path to a tiny trickle of water named Oasis Creek.

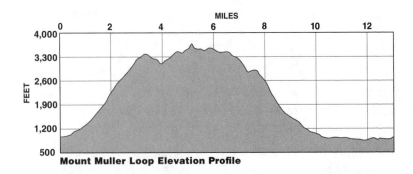

Mount Muller Loop Elevation Profile

▶**2** Except in late summer or fall, you can usually rely on a little water here, though it is always a safer bet to simply carry all you will need. Regardless of the source, you'll welcome a good drink because the climbing, and the sweating, are not yet complete.

Beyond Oasis Creek, four more winding and irregularly spaced switchbacks lead through increasingly open forests and (finally) to the ridgetop and a four-way intersection called Jim's Junction. ▶**3** Like many other named features along this loop, a small wooden sign here identifies the place. The often whimsical names for these features were bestowed by the volunteer trail crews who built this route. In most cases, the names honor their fellow crew members. (Though not, one hopes, in the case of Nosebag Point.)

At Jim's Junction, the trail to the left goes 3.7 miles to the lookout building at Kloshe Nanitch. Straight ahead is a 0.5-mile trail that descends the north side of the ridge to an isolated trailhead on a decommissioned logging road. You go right and begin the promised excellent ridge walk. The fun starts almost immediately because in just 80 yards you reach a fine rocky viewpoint where you can look down to US 101 and off to snowy Mount Olympus.

The trail now follows the sometimes narrow east–west ridgeline going in and out of forest and providing a seemingly endless array of marvelous views. In June, wildflowers—such as bear grass, bunchberry, avalanche lily, yellow violet, lupine, wild strawberry, wallflower, salmonberry, paint-brush, kinnikinnick, and many others—add color to the scenery. Over the next couple of miles, the ridge's up-and-down course takes you past signed features, such as Millsap Meadow, a low point in the ridge called Thomas Gap, particularly fetching Jasmine's Meadow, and small Allison's Meadow. At a prominent turn in the trail in Jasmine's Meadow, a brand-new trail takes off downhill and to

 Viewpoint

 Wildflowers

the right on its way back to the trailhead. This provides a good return route if you want a shorter hike.

The main trail goes straight through Jasmine's Meadow and, after completing a tiring little uphill, reaches an unnamed (or at least unsigned) meadow and a junction at 5.2 miles. Here, a trail angles left (uphill) and in 0.1 mile switchbacks three times to reach the partly forested summit of Mount Muller. ▶4 There is a partially obstructed but still decent view here to the north over the shimmering blue waters of the Strait of Juan de Fuca to Vancouver Island.

Summit

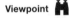
Viewpoint

If you want to slightly shorten your day, you can turn around at Mount Muller and return to your car. It is only 2.4 miles longer, however, to do the full loop, and the extra energy is well rewarded. So come back down 0.1 mile from the summit and continue hiking east on the loop trail. After only 0.1 mile, you round a corner and are presented with your first of many good views down to long and large Lake Crescent. The trail then passes signed Balance Rock (nothing much balancing here, but there are some really nice views) and several other impressive rock outcrops that aren't honored with names.

Viewpoint

Geologic Interest

The trail now includes noticeably more downhill than up as it snakes along the ridge, occasionally employing short switchbacks but mostly traversing on hillsides either in forest or in delightful rocky meadows. At 7.3 miles (including the side trip to the summit) is Cahill's Overlook, ▶5 which has nice views that seem to go straight down to US 101.

Viewpoint

A few more downhill switchbacks and you reach Mosley Gap, which at about 2,800 feet is the lowest point along the ridge. Not quite 0.3 mile later, the trail switchbacks to the right and begins a long downhill. After 25 switchbacks in just 1.3 miles, watch carefully for a small brown sign announcing the short side trail that goes left to Fout's Rock House. ▶6 Take a few minutes to investigate this site where two enormous boulders are jammed together. One of the

Geologic Interest

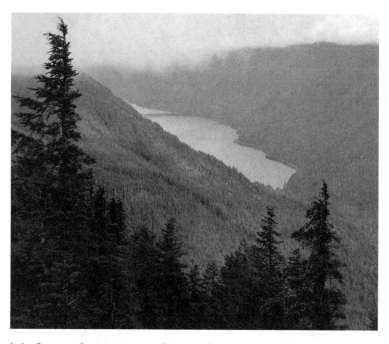

Lake Crescent *from viewpoint east of Mount Muller*

rocks is tilted at an angle that creates a large natural arch between the boulders.

About 0.25 mile below the turnoff to Fout's Rock House is an unsigned junction with a new trail that goes to the left. This path goes east to Fairholm Campground on Lake Crescent and is part of the still-in-development Olympic Discovery Trail, which is eventually scheduled to connect all the way to Port Angeles. You keep straight, pass a large spring, and continue winding your way downhill past a large gravel pit and along the hillside above US 101. At 10 miles, you hop over pretty little Hutch Creek. ▶7

The final part of the hike is less interesting and less scenic than the upper parts of the loop, as you stay nearly level in the low-elevation forests never far from US 101. In addition to the sounds of traffic,

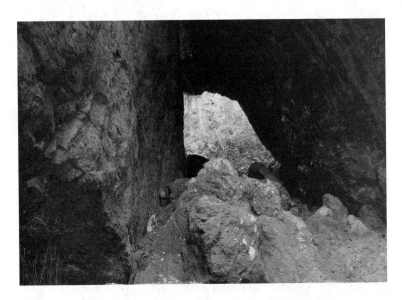

Arch *in Fout's Rock House*

other unnatural intrusions include a private home and a gravel road ►8 that you cross at 11.8 miles. The forest you are hiking through, however, is both wild and pleasant, with lots of lush vegetation, some interesting boggy places, and an abundance of songbirds in early summer. At 13 miles, you reach a junction with the brand-new trail coming down from Jasmine's Meadow and a few yards later return to the trailhead ►9 at the close of the loop.

Birds

🚶	**MILESTONES**	
►1	0.0	Trailhead (N48° 04.552' W124° 00.784')
►2	2.2	Oasis Creek (N48° 05.431' W124° 01.234')
►3	3.0	Jim's Junction (N48° 05.615' W124° 01.343')
►4	5.3	Summit of Mount Muller (N48° 05.389' W123° 58.769')
►5	7.3	Cahill's Overlook (N48° 05.472' W123° 57.275')
►6	9.0	Fout's Rock House (N48° 05.119' W123° 57.238')
►7	10.0	Hutch Creek (N48° 04.750' W123° 57.855')
►8	11.8	Gravel road (N48° 04.516' W123° 58.662')
►9	13.0	Return to trailhead (N48° 04.552' W124° 00.784')

Sol Duc Falls–Lover's Lane Loop

Most people who visit Sol Duc Falls do so by walking the short, mostly level, 0.8-mile path from the huge parking area at the end of the paved road through Sol Duc Valley. But for the dedicated pedestrian, that is a rather unsatisfying jaunt that hardly seems worthy of even being called a hike. After all, on such a short walk you never really get the chance to fully appreciate your natural surroundings, to change your mind-set from one of driving a car to one of self-propelled locomotion, or even to feel like you have really "earned" the destination at all. And besides, hiking is an activity that is at least as much about the journey itself as it is about the destination. It is much better, therefore, for both body *and* soul, to take this longer and infinitely more satisfying loop hike to the same destination. This way you enjoy more solitude; have the opportunity to see additional waterfalls, some lovely forests, and some good river views; and can more fully appreciate the wonders of this primeval environment.

Sunny skies are not necessary to enjoy this outing. In fact, this is a particularly good hiking choice for a cloudy or even a rainy day. You won't miss any views, the dark forest takes on a brooding *Lord of the Rings* sort of feeling that is surprisingly alluring, and the weather will deter the crowds that often congregate around the falls.

Best Time

The trail is usually open all year. The scenery is most attractive mid-April–early June when the forest wildflowers are blooming, the falls are full of spring

TRAIL USE
Day hiking,
child-friendly

LENGTH
5.9 miles, 3 hours

CUMULATIVE ELEVATION
450'

DIFFICULTY
- 1 **2** 3 4 5 +

TRAIL TYPE
Loop

SURFACE TYPE
Dirt, gravel

CONTOUR MAP
Green Trails *Mt Tom* #133 or Custom Correct *Seven Lakes Basin–Hoh*

START & END
N47° 58.163'
W123° 51.823'

FEATURES
Dense forest,
impressive waterfall,
beautiful river

FACILITIES
Water, resort,
hot springs

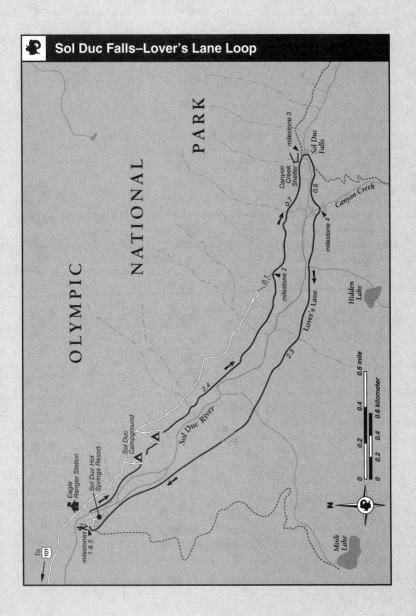

Sol Duc Falls–Lover's Lane Loop

OLYMPIC NATIONAL PARK

Eagle Ranger Station

Sol Duc Hot Springs Resort

Sol Duc Campground

milestones 1 & 5

To 101

Sol Duc River

2.4

0.1

milestone 2

0.7

Canyon Creek Shelter

milestone 3

Sol Duc Falls

0.5

Canyon Creek

milestone 4

Lover's Lane

2.3

Hidden Lake

Mink Lake

N

0 0.2 0.4 0.6 mile

0 0.2 0.4 0.6 kilometer

runoff, and the forest is bursting with new greenery. Autumn is also pleasant, when the lower water
levels make the falls more delicate and particularly
photogenic. Regardless of your seasonal timing, try
to visit on a weekday to reduce the crowds around
the falls. Or visit on a rainy or cloudy day.

Finding the Trail

Drive US 101 about 29 miles west of Port Angeles
to milepost 219.2 and a well-signed junction with
the road to Sol Duc Valley. Turn south, pass an
entrance station/fee booth just 0.3 mile later, and
proceed another 12.1 miles on this winding paved
road to a signed junction with the side road to Sol
Duc Hot Springs Resort. Turn right (toward the
resort), cross a bridge over the Sol Duc River, and
drive 0.1 mile to the signed hiker parking lot west
of the resort building and directly across from the
resort's overnight cabins.

Trail Description

You begin by backtracking from the parking area ▶1
along the access road and recrossing the road bridge
over the Sol Duc River. Immediately on the other
(north) side of this span, you turn right (upstream)
onto a wide gravel path. In very short order, this
trail passes the resort's RV parking lot/campground,
skirts a larger parking lot, and comes to the road
for Loop A in the National Park Service's inviting
Sol Duc Campground. The trail follows the campground's paved loop road for about 150 yards and
then leaves this road at a trail sign indicating that Sol
Duc Falls is 3 miles away (it's actually closer to 2.6,
but who's counting).

You turn onto this path, which takes you through
a lush, dense forest for a little more than 0.1 mile to
the road for Loop B in the campground. Keep right

Old-Growth Forest

and once again follow a paved road for about 100 yards to the signed resumption of the foot trail. The wide and gentle trail now takes you through a stately forest of moss-draped Douglas-firs and western hemlocks. The tree trunks are up to 8 feet in diameter—certainly huge, though not by comparison to some of the trees in other parts of the Olympic Peninsula—and they are impressively tall and straight. The

Birds

"music" from the nearby Sol Duc River can be heard on your right as the songs of varied thrushes, winter wrens, Swainson's thrushes, and other birds erupt from all parts of the surrounding forest. Occasionally, you may also hear the sounds of cars on the road not far to your left.

At one point, the trail veers over next to the Sol Duc River, allowing you to better appreciate this exceptionally clear stream and perhaps watch for migrating salmon. Even though you are clearly heading upstream, the trail is never steep and, in fact, the elevation gain is rarely noticeable.

At 2.4 miles, you come to a junction ▶2 with the very popular trail that starts at a road-end parking lot a little more than 0.1 mile to the left. Go right here, and temporarily say goodbye to seclusion as you follow other hikers on a wide, mostly gravel trail that goes slightly uphill in a series of intermittent stairsteps. You take a bridge over a tumbling seasonal side creek, after which the trail generally

Old-Growth Forest

levels out and travels through a cathedral forest with a particular abundance of ferns on the forest floor. About 0.7 mile from the junction is a fork in the trail immediately in front of the historic Canyon Creek

Historic Interest

Trail Shelter. This lovely log structure is well worth investigating and even has a covered wooden veranda to protect hikers from the rain.

You go right at the fork and just 40 yards later come to a bridge over the Sol Duc River immediately

Waterfall

downstream from beautiful Sol Duc Falls. ▶3 Here, the river divides into between two and four adjacent falls (depending on water levels) that drop into a narrow and dark canyon. The dramatic falls, along with the lovely forest setting, makes this location exceptionally photogenic, especially when viewed from the bridge. During the high runoff of spring and early summer, you can expect to get wet from the spray from the falls, which is very refreshing on a hot day. If you turn around and look downstream from the bridge, you'll have a fine view of the river as it charges through a narrow chasm. Once across the wooden bridge, check out another excellent fenced-in viewing area, which is just on the upstream side of the trail.

After fully enjoying the falls, turn downstream and walk about 0.1 mile to a junction. For the loop hike, turn right on Lover's Lane Trail, a gentle and woodsy path that, as the name suggests, is ideal for quiet strolling by lovers or anyone else. The first 0.1 mile of this path offers some nice views down into the Sol Duc River's deep chasm. Don't be too distracted by the fine forest and river scenery, however, because the path also contains a fair number of roots and rocks that present a tripping hazard.

About 0.4 mile along Lover's Lane is a log bridge over good-size Canyon Creek. ►4 Immediately downstream from the bridge is a crashing segmented waterfall. A scramble trail down the east side of the creek provides a partially obstructed view of this tall cascade. A somewhat shorter but still very pretty falls can be found about 60 yards upstream from the bridge.

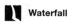 **Waterfall**

Over the next 0.3 mile, you pass a few small intermittent creeks, and then the trail crosses river-level flats with big and relatively widely spaced trees and lush undergrowth. In the spring, white-blooming Unalaska bunchberry, vanilla leaf, Pacific trillium, American starflower, and Siberian spring beauty, as well as lavender-colored Pacific bleeding heart, add colors other than green to the scene. The

 Wildflowers

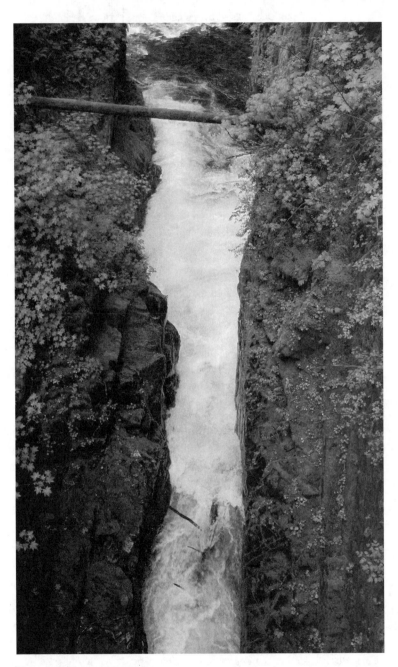

Slot canyon *below Sol Duc Falls*

hiking remains very easy for the rest of the way and even includes a short boardwalk over a particularly boggy section to keep your feet dry and clean. Eventually, your nose will pick up an increasingly strong sulfur smell as you approach and then walk past the swimming pools of the Sol Duc Hot Springs Resort. Just 0.1 mile later is a junction with Mink Lake Trail. You go right and walk a final 50 yards to the trailhead parking area. ▶5

🚶 MILESTONES

▶1	0.0	Parking lot west of Sol Duc Hot Spring Resort (N47° 47.972' W123° 57.261')
▶2	2.4	Junction (N47° 57.214' W123° 49.977')
▶3	3.1	Sol Duc Falls (N47° 57.215' W123° 49.982')
▶4	3.6	Canyon Creek (N47° 57.048' W123° 49.608')
▶5	5.9	Return to trailhead (N47° 47.972' W123° 57.261')

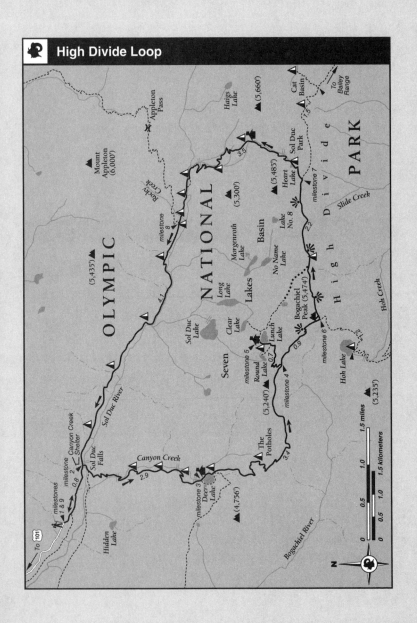

High Divide Loop

On maintained trails in the Olympic Mountains, not much really compares to High Divide. Here, the views are arguably better, the wildlife more abundant, the flowers more numerous, the lakes more common, and the scenery unsurpassed. If you only have time for one overnight hike in the Olympic Mountains, then this should be it. Of course, lots of other people agree with this assessment, so don't expect solitude.

Wildlife (especially black bears) is common. I suppose it is possible to spend a full day hiking during the late summer and early fall berry season on the High Divide and *not* see a bear, but in my several visits here over the years, that is a trick I have never managed to pull. On one memorable day, the bruins seemed to be around every corner, and I spotted a total of 14 of them! So keep your eyes open, both for the thrill of seeing impressive wildlife and to avoid the very rare, but potentially dangerous, circumstance where you end up surprising a sow black bear with cubs. Because of the bears, the National Park Service requires that all overnight visitors use a bear canister. If you do not own one, they are available for rent from the ranger station when you pick up your permit.

To protect this popular area, the NPS has developed a limited number of designated campsites and employs a reservation system for overnight hiking between May 1 and September 30. Approximately half of the available camping spots are given out in reserved permits, with the remainder offered on a first-come, first-serve basis. To apply for a reservation, visit the park's website (**nps.gov/olym**),

TRAIL USE
Backpacking, horses
LENGTH
20.3 miles (including recommended side trips to Lunch Lake and Bogachiel Peak), 2–3 days
CUMULATIVE ELEVATION
5,200' (with side trips)
DIFFICULTY
- 1 2 3 4 **5** +
TRAIL TYPE
Loop
SURFACE TYPE
Dirt, gravel
CONTOUR MAP
Custom Correct *Seven Lakes Basin–Hoh*
START & END
N47° 57.297'
W123° 50.092'

FEATURES
Mountain views, abundant wildlife (especially bears), wildflowers, mountain lakes

FACILITIES
Restrooms, picnic tables

download a Wilderness Camping Permit Reservation Request form, fill out your information and planned itinerary, include your payment, and then send it by snail mail or fax (360-565-3108) to the Wilderness Information Center.

Best Time

The trail is usually open late July–mid-October. Frequently, however, deep snows remain on the north sides of ridges and in Seven Lakes Basin well into August. The trip is good (make that spectacular) any time it is open, but it's especially appealing in late July and August, when the wildflowers are blooming. Late summer and early fall are best for wildlife viewing. Good weather is a must because you really don't want to miss the views.

Finding the Trail

Drive US 101 about 29 miles west of Port Angeles to milepost 219.2 and a well-signed junction with the road to Sol Duc Valley. Turn south, pass an entrance station/fee booth just 0.3 mile later, and proceed another 13.8 miles on this winding paved road to the large (but nonetheless often full) road-end parking lot and trailhead.

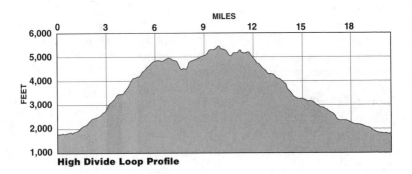

High Divide Loop Profile

Trail Description

Go east from the parking lot ►1 on the well-signed
and heavily used Sol Duc Trail, which takes you
through a stately and impressive forest of big old
Douglas-firs and western hemlocks. The gravel path
is wide and gentle with only minor ups and downs.
At a little more than 0.1 mile is a junction with a
trail that comes up from Sol Duc Campground and
serves as the northern half of the Lover's Lane Loop
(Trail 14). Go straight on the main trail, enjoying
not only the sights of this fine forest but its sounds
as well: the calls of jays and thrushes, the distant
rumble of the river, and the sound of wind in the
trees. You cross a few small creeks on wooden
bridges and then at 0.8 mile come to a fork in the
trail in front of the log Canyon Creek Shelter. This
is the start of the loop.

**Old-Growth
Forest**

Go right at this junction and immediately drop
to a bridge over the river just below crashing Sol
Duc Falls. ►2 This dramatic multisectioned falls
drops into a fern-filled slot canyon and is understandably one of the most photographed trailside
locations in the park. Most hikers turn around at
this point and return to their cars. There is a great
view of the falls from the bridge and another good
viewing area at a log-lined overlook on the south
side of the crossing. Expect to get wet from spray
produced by the falls.

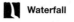

Waterfall

The rocky trail curves a little to the right (downstream) from the bridge and in 0.1 mile reaches
a junction with Lover's Lane Trail (Trail 14). Go
straight (uphill) and begin your climb toward the
high country. For the next mile or two, the trail is
rather eroded and frequently resembles a dry creek
bed with lots of rocks and log steps for the non-
existent water to cascade over. Without question,
you are heading "upstream" as you steadily gain
elevation. A few scattered switchbacks keep the

Steep

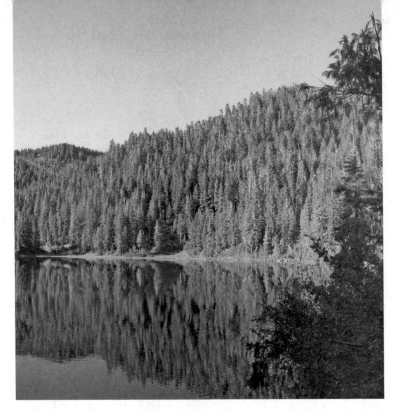

Deer Lake

grade relatively moderate, but you'll still need plenty of rest breaks as you lug the heavy pack uphill.

You soon enter the canyon of Canyon Creek and for the next couple of miles follow that clear, cascading stream. You cross the creek on a wooden bridge directly over a deep chasm and waterfall and then ascend the west side of the canyon, still in mostly viewless forest. About 0.4 mile above the bridge, you pass Canyon Creek Campsite 1, the first designated camp for those who got a late start. Even nicer Canyon Creek Campsite 2 comes along less than a mile later. More winding uphill takes you to a pretty waterfall on Canyon Creek, though it requires a bit of scrambling to get a decent view.

Waterfall

Waterfall

At a switchback just above this falls, you pass a spur trail to a third campsite at a sign saying that open fires are prohibited beyond this point. Another hard-to-see waterfall comes along just before you reach tranquil and forest-rimmed Deer Lake. ►3 A side trail goes to the right here around the lake's west side, but the main trail heads to the left, crossing a bridge over Canyon Creek where it leaves the lake. This path passes side trails to designated campsites, toilets, and a seasonal ranger station before reaching a reunion with the loop trail around the west side of the lake.

 Waterfall

 Lake

Just beyond this junction is a possibly unsigned fork. The route to Little Divide and Mink Lake goes right, but you keep left and soon pass a dark little pond surrounded by trees and heather meadows. Look for deer here, especially in the morning, and expect lots of mosquitoes. As you continue climbing, you'll notice that the forest is much more open now and is dominated by higher-elevation conifers such as Alaska yellow cedar, Pacific silver fir, and mountain hemlock. The understory is mostly bear grass, heather, and huckleberry—the last offering up delicious treats in late summer and early fall. Bears love these berries too, so don't be surprised to round a corner and see a bruin. Less than a mile above Deer Lake, you pass a relatively flat area that is sometimes referred to as The Potholes because the meadow here is sprinkled with a dozen or so scenic tarns. A couple of nice designated campsites allow you to linger overnight in this pretty area, though you should expect mosquitoes.

 Wildlife

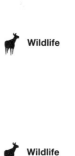 **Wildlife**

Lake

Now you ascend a set of 10 switchbacks that take you up through increasingly open terrain and fields of white, July-blooming avalanche lilies to the top of High Divide. At first, you can't see much of anything as you walk on a nearly level trail through forest. Things improve markedly, however, when you leave the forest and round the scenic basin at the headwaters of the Bogachiel River. This basin is rimmed with jagged, snow-streaked

Wildflowers

Viewpoint 🔭 crags and offers excellent views down the long, forested canyon of this wilderness river. You then go through a little saddle on the north side of High Divide and cross a rocky area to a junction with the Seven Lakes Basin Trail. ▶4

The main loop trail goes straight, but the Seven Lakes Basin, with its (more than seven) beautiful lakes, idyllic meadows, and superb campsites is to the left. You'll want to at least explore this delightful basin and possibly spend a night here, so turn left and descend a half dozen switchbacks into the basin. At the bottom is a junction with the 0.15-mile downhill spur trail to Round Lake, which is

Lake 〰️ also well worth a visit. The main trail goes straight and soon deposits you on the shores of wonderfully scenic Lunch Lake, ▶5 which is backed by the hulking flank of Bogachiel Peak. Posted maps and signs direct you through the myriad of trails and designated campsites near this very popular lake. There is also a seasonal ranger station and a privy. You won't have the place to yourself, but this is still a wonderful location to spend a night in the wilderness. If you want to do some exploring, side trails lead down to Clear Lake to the north and up to a pair of gorgeous unnamed ponds to the southeast. These ponds typically remain at least partially ice-bound until early August.

Back at the junction on High Divide, you go east, traverse the south side of the ridge for about 0.3 mile, and then make six short uphill switchbacks to the top of the divide. The next 100 yards or so on the north side of the ridge are often covered with steep snow until late summer, causing a problem for hikers, especially on cold or icy mornings.

Once back on the south side of the divide, you traverse an open slope, passing an unsigned but obvious junction with an unofficial use trail up the west side of Bogachiel Peak. Keep straight and come to a saddle where there is a junction with the trail to Hoh Lake. ▶6

You keep left here, staying on the High Divide Trail, and ascend for 0.2 mile to a junction with the official 0.15-mile trail to the top of Bogachiel Peak. It's well worth the minimal effort to reach this former lookout site; it offers excellent views back down to Lunch Lake and the Seven Lakes Basin, as well as west to the Pacific Ocean. Dominating the view, however, both from Bogachiel Peak and the High Divide Trail in general, is the look south to the icy crags of dramatic Mount Olympus and Mount Tom. Many consider this to be the supreme view in the park. Although I can think of a few that I would rate higher, this is still outstanding, especially with the dark green of the deep and heavily forested valley of the Hoh River filling the foreground.

 Summit

 Viewpoint

The view-packed High Divide Trail now makes its way east, offering up two of the most delightful miles of hiking in the park. The views are superb; the alpine meadows and wildflowers are great; and the wildlife, especially bears and elk in the meadows of Seven Lakes Basin to your left (north), are plentiful. Occasionally, mountain goats are seen along this ridge as well. The route includes several steep little ups and downs, and you will have to negotiate a few snowfields across the route until about late July, but on balance it's a great walk.

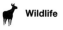 **Wildlife**

At a low point in the ridge about 0.6 mile from Bogachiel Peak, a boot path angles in from the left, coming up from Seven Lakes Basin. Keep straight on the main route and soon reach small Silver Snag Campsite. Although wildly scenic, the only available water here is from nearby snowfields that linger into early August. *Tip:* There are two other legal but hidden campsites along High Divide, but you'll need directions from a ranger to find them. It is well worth the extra effort, however, as they offer privacy and outstanding views.

Near the east end of this fun section, you pass well above the circular form of Lake No. 8 in the upper part of Seven Lakes Basin. (Yeah, I know, there shouldn't be a Lake No. 8 in a "Seven" Lakes Basin, but I didn't name these features.) You then cross over to the next basin draining north and look down on small Heart Lake, which is much better named because it closely resembles the classic Valentine's Day symbol. Soon you reach a junction.

The loop trail goes left (downhill) toward Heart Lake and Sol Duc Park. If you still have plenty of energy and a few hours of extra time, however, spend them on some additional explorations of High Divide on the trail that goes straight at this junction toward Cat Basin. This trail is mostly level for about 0.6 mile and then passes a spur trail to a very pretty but waterless campsite. From here, the route winds down mostly open slopes to a junction. The trail to the scenic stock campsite in Cat Basin goes left (downhill). For perhaps the best views on all of High Divide, however, continue straight, descend a bit, and then climb through forest for about 1.3 miles to

Viewpoint where you finally break out of the trees. Here, you are afforded absolutely breathtaking views to the south–southwest of spectacular Mount Olympus. Beyond this good turnaround point, the trail crosses the very steep slopes on the south side of Cat Peak and rapidly becomes very narrow and rather rough. Eventually, the old trail disappears entirely, leaving the rest of the route for hikers doing the long cross-country route along the Bailey Range. Those not up for this rugged weeklong adventure, however, must reluctantly turn around and return to the Sol Duc Park junction the way they came. *Tip:* This side trip makes a great day hike for those spending an extra day at a camp at Heart Lake or in Sol Duc Park.

Lake The return route of the loop descends flower-dotted open slopes for 0.4 mile to beautiful but small Heart Lake ▶7 (good campsites), and then

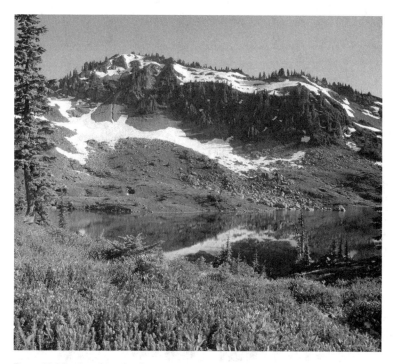

Bogachiel Peak *and Lunch Lake*

crosses its outlet creek a little below the lake. A couple of downhill switchbacks take you past a small waterfall and into a partly forested area of rolling meadowlands called Sol Duc Park. At the lower end of these parklands, you cross Bridge Creek (where, ironically, there is no bridge) and then pass several spur trails leading to designated campsites and a seasonal ranger station.

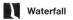 **Waterfall**

About 0.5 mile later, you cross Bridge Creek again, this time on a log bridge, at the Lower Bridge Creek Campsites. Now back in heavy forest, the often rocky trail steadily winds downhill in switchbacks and traverses. Near the bottom, you come to a fork in the trail. A stock camp and river crossing is to the left.

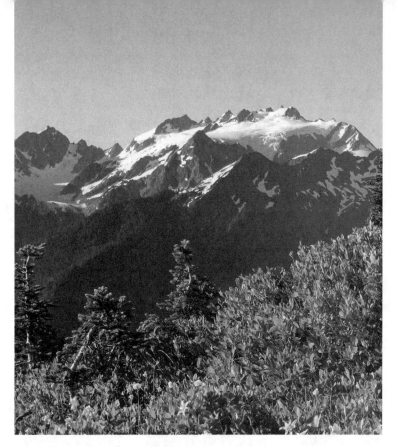

Mount Olympus *from High Divide Trail*

You veer right and drop a bit more to the shady Sol Duc Crossing Campsite and, immediately thereafter, a footlog over the loudly cascading Sol Duc River.

Now heading downstream on the north side of the river, you pass a reunion with the stock trail after 0.1 mile and a large group campsite 0.2 mile after that. Next in line are a designated campsite just before the log crossing of tumbling Rocky Creek and another one about 100 yards later at the junction with the trail to Appleton Pass. ▶8

Go straight (west) here; for the rest of the hike, travel through viewless but attractive old-growth forests. Overall, the route gradually loses elevation,

Old-Growth Forest

but it has plenty of small ups and downs along the way. Scattered along the trail are four designated campsites for those who want to experience a night in this impressive forest. The trail is only sporadically near the river, but when it is, the stream is usually rushing through a steep-walled chasm with lots of lovely cascades and small waterfalls. At 4.1 miles from the Appleton Pass turnoff, you return to the junction beside Sol Duc Falls and the Canyon Creek Shelter at the close of the loop. Go straight and retrace your route 0.8 mile to the trailhead. ►9

| 大 | **MILESTONES** |

►1	0.0	Trailhead (N47° 57.297' W123° 50.092')
►2	0.8	Sol Duc Falls (N47° 57.215' W123° 49.982')
►3	3.7	Deer Lake outlet (N47° 55.675' W123° 49.432')
►4	7.1	Seven Lakes Basin junction (N47° 54.722' W123° 47.394')
►5	7.8	Lunch Lake (N47° 54.898' W123° 47.084')
►6	9.4	Hoh Lake junction (N47° 54.255' W123° 46.692')
►7	12.3	Heart Lake (N47° 54.590' W123° 44.026')
►8	15.4	Appleton Pass junction (N47° 55.942' W123° 45.021')
►9	20.3	Return to trailhead (N47° 57.297' W123° 50.092')

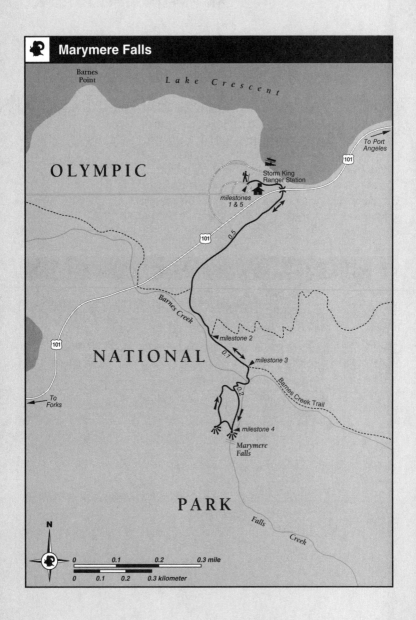

Marymere Falls

Barnes Point

Lake Crescent

OLYMPIC

To Port Angeles

101

Storm King
Ranger Station

milestones
1 & 5

101

0.5

Barnes Creek

milestone 2

NATIONAL

0.1

milestone 3

Barnes Creek Trail

101

0.2

To Forks

milestone 4

Marymere Falls

PARK

Falls Creek

N

0   0.1   0.2   0.3 mile

0   0.1   0.2   0.3 kilometer

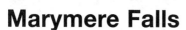

Marymere Falls

Marymere Falls is one of the most popular trail destinations in Olympic National Park. Thousands of sneaker-clad tourists trek up the easy trail to this falls, which offers them a welcome opportunity to stretch their legs. Of even greater appeal, however, is that the falls is a very beautiful and photogenic destination set in a mossy canyon where the waters of Falls Creek drop impressively over a basalt cliff and spread out in a veil at the base. You won't have this trail to yourself, but you also won't regret the relatively minimal effort required to reach this lovely spot.

Best Time

The trail is usually open all year, though the canyon can get cold and icy in the winter months. Spring offers the highest water, so the falls are more dramatic. This short hike is *extremely* popular with the summer crowds, so if you want something approaching solitude, hike on a weekday . . . in the off-season . . . while it's raining.

Finding the Trail

Drive US 101 about 20 miles west of Port Angeles along the south shore of Lake Crescent to a turnoff at milepost 227.9. Turn right (north), following signs to Storm King Ranger Station, and go 0.1 mile to a four-way junction. Turn right and come to the large parking area about 0.1 mile later.

Trail Description

Locate the signed Marymere Falls Trail next to the log Storm King Ranger Station beside the east end

TRAIL USE
Day hiking,
child-friendly

LENGTH
1.6 miles, 1 hour

**CUMULATIVE
ELEVATION**
200'

DIFFICULTY
- **1** 2 3 4 5 +

TRAIL TYPE
Out-and-back

SURFACE TYPE
Gravel, dirt

CONTOUR MAP
The map on the trail-
head signboard is
sufficient.

START & END
N48° 03.481'
W123° 47.345'

FEATURES
Beautiful lacy waterfall,
big trees, clear creeks

FACILITIES
Restrooms, picnic
tables, ranger station

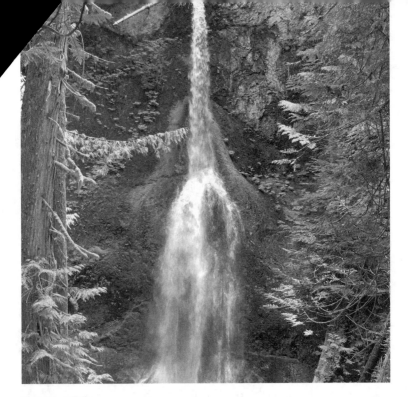

Marymere Falls

Lake

of the parking lot. ▶1 The trail is initially paved, but immediately past the ranger station building, it turns to gravel and takes you into the forest beside a boat ramp on Lake Crescent. From here, you briefly parallel the shore of the lake and then take a pedestrian tunnel under very busy US 101.

The wide and heavily used trail now angles to the right and stays close to the highway for the next 0.2 mile or so, where, despite the natural surroundings of Douglas-fir and western red cedar forest, it's impossible to escape the sound of cars. Eventually the traffic noise is replaced by the all-natural symphony of "river music" from rushing Barnes Creek on your right.

At almost 0.4 mile, a signed trail goes right toward Lake Crescent Lodge, but you keep straight and walk another 0.1 mile to the signed junction ▶2 with the steep and lesser-used trail up Mount Storm King (Trail 17). This trail, which goes up the hill to the left, is a good alternative for hikers who prefer seclusion and views, but only if they can handle a steep climb.

Marymere Falls Trail continues straight at this junction and soon takes you past some impressive old trees that are ideal for taking pictures of the kids beside these natural giants. At 0.6 mile is yet another junction, ▶3 this time with Barnes Creek Trail, which goes straight. This is another good option for solitude seekers, though it has few scenic highlights other than some pleasant old-growth forests.

Old-Growth Forest

For the main attraction, go right at this junction, still following signs to Marymere Falls, and about 100 yards later take first a bridge over large Barnes Creek and then a log span across much smaller Falls Creek. The trail now climbs a series of steps in two quick switchbacks to a junction at the start of a mini-loop up to the falls. Go left here and ascend a trail that is lined on its downhill side with a wooden fence. Falls Creek flows in the canyon below you on the left. After 0.1 mile, or not quite 0.8 mile from the trailhead, you reach a viewpoint ▶4 right across from the lovely drop of 90-foot-high Marymere Falls.

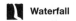
Waterfall

The return portion of the mini-loop goes sharply right at this lower viewpoint and climbs a few more stairs to a second, higher viewpoint of the falls. A little bench here allows you to admire the scene at leisure before you turn around and go steeply downhill back to the junction at the close of the mini-loop. Go straight and retrace your steps to the trailhead. ▶5

🚶	**MILESTONES**	
▶1	0.0	Take trail from parking lot (N48° 03.481' W123° 47.345')
▶2	0.5	Mount Storm King junction (N48° 03.214' W123° 47.401')
▶3	0.6	Barnes Creek Trail junction (N48° 03.127' W123° 47.272')
▶4	0.8	Marymere Falls viewpoint (N48° 03.039' W123° 47.313')
▶5	1.6	Return to trailhead (N48° 03.481' W123° 47.345')

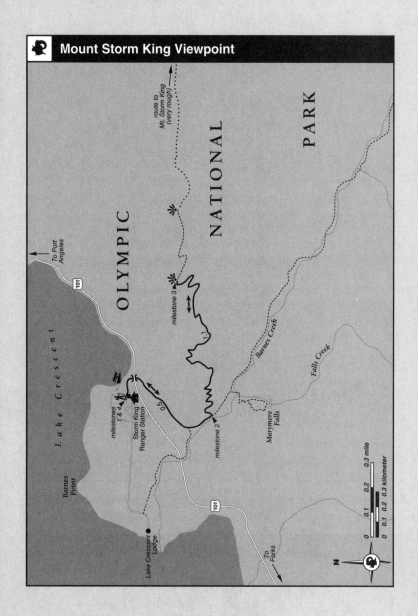

Mount Storm King Viewpoint

route to
Mt. Storm King
(very rough)

NATIONAL

PARK

OLYMPIC

To Port
Angeles

101

Lake Crescent

milestone 3

Barnes Creek

Falls Creek

Barnes
Point

0.5

milestones
1 & 4

Storm King
Ranger Station

milestone 2

Marymere
Falls

Lake Crescent
Lodge

101

To
Forks

0   0.1   0.2   0.3 mile

0   0.1   0.2   0.3 kilometer

N

Mount Storm King Viewpoint

Unless you happen to be a bald eagle, the best bird's-eye view of Lake Crescent is from a trailside outlook partway up Mount Storm King. Unfortunately, reaching this observation point is a whole lot easier for eagles than it is for humans. Without the "unfair" advantage of feathers, we are forced to envy the avians as we trudge up a steep and tiring trail to reach the same perspective that they acquire with just a few flaps of their giant wings. On the plus side, the trail is fairly short and mostly in the shade, though it's still a good idea to hike in the cool of the morning rather than the heat of a summer afternoon.

Best Time

The trail is usually open from about April to mid-November. Save this hike for a nice day to fully appreciate the views. Mornings are preferable, so you can hike in the cooler hours of the day.

Finding the Trail

Drive US 101 about 20 miles west of Port Angeles along the south shore of Lake Crescent to a turnoff at milepost 227.9. Turn right (north), following signs to Storm King Ranger Station, and go 0.1 mile to a four-way junction. Turn right and come to the large parking area about 0.1 mile later.

TRAIL USE
Day hiking

LENGTH
3.2 miles, 2.5 hours

**CUMULATIVE
ELEVATION**
1,460'

DIFFICULTY
- 1 2 **3** 4 5 +

TRAIL TYPE
Out-and-back

SURFACE TYPE
Gravel, dirt

CONTOUR MAP
Custom Correct *Lake
Crescent–Happy
Lake Ridge*

START & END
N48° 03.481'
W123° 47.345'

FEATURES
Views of large Lake
Crescent, diverse
forests

FACILITIES
Restrooms, picnic
tables, ranger station

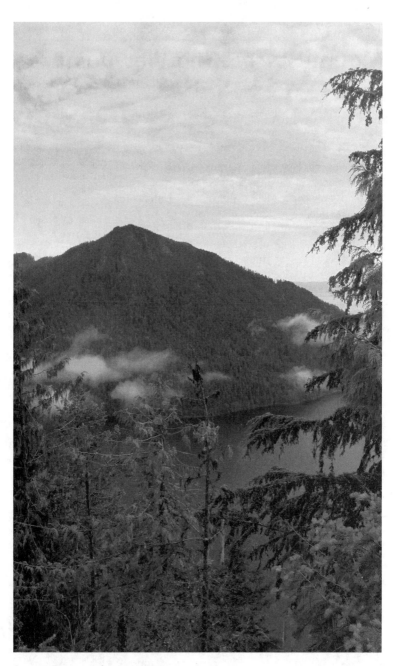

Pyramid Mountain *from Mount Storm King Viewpoint*

Trail Description

The signed Marymere Falls Trail begins next to the log Storm King Ranger Station at the east end of the parking lot. ▶1 The trail is initially paved but soon turns to gravel as it enters the forest along the shore of Lake Crescent and passes through a pedestrian tunnel under US 101. The wide, almost level, and heavily used trail now angles to the right, staying close to the unseen but easily heard highway for the next 0.2 mile. After almost 0.4 mile, a signed trail goes right toward Lake Crescent Lodge, but you keep straight, soon leaving the sounds of the highway behind.

 Lake

At just under 0.5 mile is a junction ▶2 beside an enormous, house-size boulder on the left side of the trail with a small, brown sign saying STORM KING TRAIL. You turn left here and immediately begin the hard part of this hike, a steep and steady climb in a series of switchbacks. Initially, you are in dense and viewless forest, but things dry out and open up as you ascend. The forest changes from big old Douglas-firs and western hemlocks to a mix of Pacific madrone trees with more widely scattered Douglas-firs and western red cedars. The more-open forest provides partial views, but on the other hand there is less shade, so the hike can be uncomfortably hot on summer afternoons.

 Steep

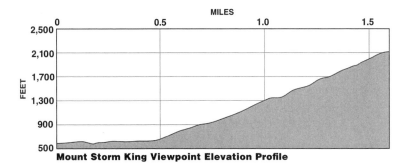

Mount Storm King Viewpoint Elevation Profile

After eight switchbacks, you come to a very small flat area with what looks like an old campsite on your left. Stop to catch your breath here because this flat spot only lasts for about 30 yards before it's back to the steep climb, now in longer switchbacks and traverses. A couple of nice views of the Barnes Creek valley and surrounding ridges offer rewards along the way and a good excuse to stop and rest.

Viewpoint 📷

After a final set of four somewhat shorter switchbacks, you reach the promised viewpoint. ▶3 Perched on a narrow rocky ledge (watch your step!), this outlook offers a breathtaking scene as you peer seemingly straight down to the deep blue water of enormous Lake Crescent. Across the lake is aptly named Pyramid Mountain, and you can even look beyond that to the Strait of Juan de Fuca and Vancouver Island. It's not a place for those afraid of heights, but it is certainly a great spot for lovers of fine viewpoints. Although the trail keeps climbing from here, this ledge offers the best panoramas of the lake. *Note:* Be very careful on the way back down to the trailhead ▶4 because there are a couple of steep sections with loose pebbles and rocks, which offer poor footing and could lead to a fall.

🚶 MILESTONES

▶1	0.0	Take trail from ranger station (N48° 03.481' W123° 47.345')
▶2	0.5	Junction (N48° 03.214' W123° 47.401')
▶3	1.6	Ledge viewpoint (N48° 03.322' W123° 46.741')
▶4	3.2	Return to trailhead (N48° 03.481' W123° 47.345')

Spruce Railroad Trail

During World War I, the strong and lightweight wood of Sitka spruce was considered an ideal material for manufacturing a newfangled machine with potential military applications known as an airplane. (You may have heard about them.) To collect this wood, a railroad was built on the northern Olympic Peninsula from the lumber mills at Port Angeles to the forests where the trees grew. The war ended just as construction was completed, but the railroad was still used for general logging purposes for several decades. Today, a portion of the old railroad bed has been converted into an extremely scenic trail along the north shore of Lake Crescent. In addition to offering frequent views of this enormous lake, the hiking is remarkably easy because the old railroad bed is nearly level. Unlike almost every other trail in Olympic National Park, this path is open to a wide variety of users, including horses, mountain bikes, and dogs, so this is an excellent option for visitors with pets or those who prefer a different form of transport than walking. *Note:* As of this writing, the National Park Service is planning to upgrade this historic route to make it wheelchair-accessible along the entire trail. They also want to upgrade bridges, reopen old railroad tunnels, and generally improve the tread throughout. This process is scheduled to begin in 2014 and may take several years and could involve periodic closures of the trail for construction. Call ahead about the latest conditions.

Best Time

The trail is usually open all year, though a few times each winter, low-elevation snow and ice may

TRAIL USE
Day hiking, mountain biking, horses, dogs allowed, child-friendly

LENGTH
5.8 miles, 3 hours

CUMULATIVE ELEVATION
250'

DIFFICULTY
- 1 **2** 3 4 5 +

TRAIL TYPE
Out-and-back (or point to point with car shuttle)

SURFACE TYPE
Gravel, dirt

CONTOUR MAP
Custom Correct *Lake Crescent–Happy Lake Ridge*

START & END
N48° 05.602'
W123° 48.148'

FEATURES
Views across large and clear Lake Crescent, historical interest

FACILITIES
Restrooms, picnic tables

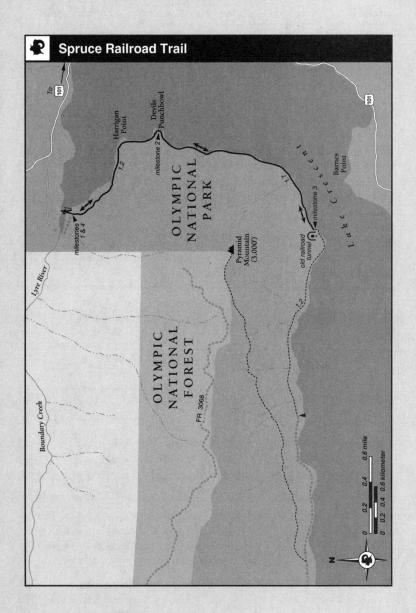

Spruce Railroad Trail

To 113

Harrigan Point

Devils Punchbowl

milestone 2

OLYMPIC NATIONAL PARK

Lake Crescent

Barnes Point

.1

milestone 3

old railroad tunnel

.1

milestones 1 & 4

Lyre River

Pyramid Mountain (3,000')

.2

OLYMPIC NATIONAL FOREST

FR 3068

Boundary Creek

0   0.2   0.4   0.6 mile
0   0.2   0.4   0.6 kilometer

N

temporarily close the trail or access road. Good weather isn't required but is preferable to enjoy the fine views across the lake to the surrounding ridges. Wildflowers peak in May or early June.

Finding the Trail

Drive US 101 about 15.5 miles west of Port Angeles to milepost 232 and a well-signed junction. Turn right (northwest) on East Beach Road, a narrow paved road that winds past small homes along the northeast shore of Lake Crescent. After 3.4 miles, just after passing the turnoff to Log Cabin Resort, you turn left at a junction, following signs to Spruce Railroad Trail. Drive 0.7 mile to a bridge over Lyre River (the outlet to Lake Crescent), and then proceed on what now turns to a gravel road for a final 0.15 mile to the marked trailhead on the left. *Note:* Do *not* park or drive past the trailhead, as it immediately becomes a private road/driveway.

Trail Description

The gravel path departs on the south side of the road, opposite the lake and the trailhead parking lot, ▶1 climbing gently through an open and exceptionally attractive second-growth forest. Widely spaced Douglas-firs, western red cedars, and big-leaf maples are the largest living things in these parts, while sword and bracken ferns and various grasses carpet the forest floor. After skirting some inholdings of private property, the trail descends back down to the old railroad bed near the lake and remains there for the rest of the hike. Views of the water are hit and miss through the trees, but they are still good, and it is well worth scrambling out on any of several unmarked boot paths to get an even better look. Lake Crescent is one of the deepest (up to 600 feet) and purest large natural lakes in

 Lake

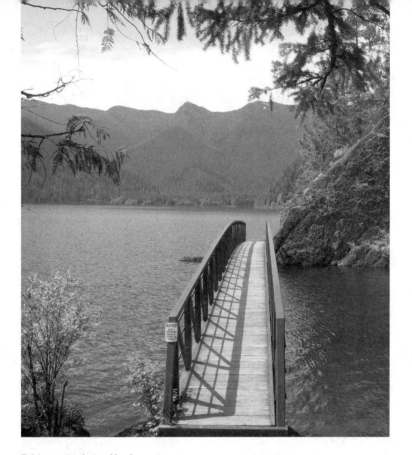

Bridge *at Devils Punchbowl*

Washington and is surrounded by attractive ridges that are heavily blanketed with forest. Boaters can see more than 40 feet down into the clear waters, and the fishing is often excellent.

At just more than 1.2 miles, you reach the picturesque bridge across Devils Punchbowl, ▶2 a very deep little inlet where you can look down into the amazingly clear water and see schools of silvery fish. Photogenic rocks and Pacific madrone trees frame fine views across the lake from here to the nearby ridges. In May and June the bright yellow blossoms of stonecrop growing in the cracks of the rocks add color to the wonderful scene.

Viewpoint

Wildflowers 🌸

Beyond Devils Punchbowl, the nearly level old railroad route continues to hug the shoreline, sometimes amid the trees and sometimes on open rocky slopes right above the water where you will gather inspiring views. At about 2.9 miles, you come to an old railroad tunnel ▶3 that as of 2014 was blocked off by a tumble of rocks and debris. The trail skirts around this old tunnel on the left (lake) side of the rock. As part of the planned upgrading of this trail, the National Park Service hopes to reopen this tunnel for travelers to pass through it.

Because you have just finished walking the trail's most attractive section, this tunnel makes a logical turnaround point for this trip, so return to the trailhead ▶4 the way you came.

If you have two cars, or just want more exercise, you can keep going another 1.2 miles to the trail's western terminus. To reach this point by car, return to US 101 and drive west to a junction at milepost 221. Turn right (north) onto Camp David Junior Road and proceed on this initially paved and then narrow gravel road for 5 miles to the small parking lot and trailhead at road-end.

 Viewpoint

 Historic Interest

🚶	**MILESTONES**	
▶1	0.0	Take trail from parking area (N48° 05.602' W123° 48.148')
▶2	1.2	Devils Punchbowl (N48° 04.986' W123° 47.263')
▶3	2.9	Old railroad tunnel (N48° 03.897' W123° 48.260')
▶4	5.8	Return to trailhead (N48° 05.602' W123° 48.148')

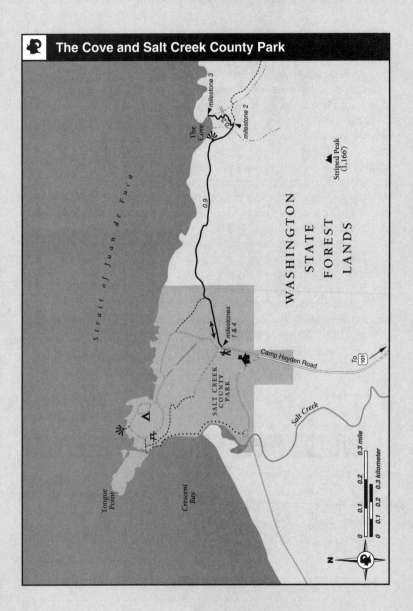

milestone 3

The Cove

milestone 2

0.2

Striped Peak
(1,166')

0.9

Strait of Juan de Fuca

WASHINGTON
STATE
FOREST
LANDS

milestones
1 & 4

SALT CREEK COUNTY PARK

Camp Hayden Road

To 101

Salt Creek

Tongue
Point

Crescent
Bay

0.3 mile

0   0.1   0.2   0.3 kilometer

N

The Cove and Salt Creek County Park

Even though I obviously haven't checked out all county parks in the country, Salt Creek County Park has to be one of the nicest. Though well known by locals, very few visitors to the region have ever even heard about the park, and fewer still take the time to see it for themselves. That is a big mistake because there is a lot to see and do here, including spotting the dozens of deer that often graze in a large meadow in the middle of the park; staying overnight at the very comfortable campground; having lunch at the park's superb picnic areas; taking in the excellent views across the Strait of Juan de Fuca; exploring the beaches of Crescent Bay (one of the best on the Olympic Peninsula); photographing the small islands and offshore rocks that provide plenty of scenic interest; and, perhaps best of all, checking out the extensive area of tidepools that offer some of the best of this sport you will find anywhere. There are options for the hiker here as well, with short strolls around Crescent Bay and the tidepool areas near Tongue Point, and a longer trail that starts in the park and soon enters adjacent Washington Department of Natural Resources land on its way to a viewpoint on Striped Peak. The trail all the way to the top is interesting and the views are pretty good, though nothing that you would call outstanding (at least not for this region). The shorter and more interesting option recommended here is to only go part of the way along Striped Peak Trail, and then leave that route for a little-used side path that drops to a tiny hidden ocean inlet, rather prosaically called The Cove. This spot is not only very pretty,

TRAIL USE
Day hiking, dogs allowed, child-friendly

LENGTH
2.2 miles (to The Cove; plus as much exploring in other areas of the park as you want), 2 hours

CUMULATIVE ELEVATION
400'

DIFFICULTY
- 1 **2** 3 4 5 +

TRAIL TYPE
Out-and-back

SURFACE TYPE
Dirt, gravel

CONTOUR MAP
None needed

START & END
N48° 09.738'
W123° 41.909'
(for The Cove hike)

FEATURES
Tidepooling, coastal scenery, photogenic beach

FACILITIES
Water, picnic areas, campground, restrooms

but there is also an excellent chance that you will
have it all to yourself.

Best Time

The park and trail are usually open all year. Low tide
is not required but is preferable because it allows for
greater access and for lots of fun tidepool exploring,
especially around Tongue Point and Crescent Bay.

Finding the Trail

Drive US 101 about 5 miles west of Port Angeles
to milepost 242.6 and a junction with Washington
Highway 112. Turn west onto this highway, following signs to Neah Bay and Sekiu, drive 7.4 miles,
and then turn right on Camp Hayden Road. After
3.6 miles, you come to a fork. The left branch goes
to Crescent Bay, which is well worth exploring. The
right fork goes 0.1 mile to the turnoff to the small
parking area for Striped Peak Trailhead on the right.
This is also the starting point for the trail to The Cove.

To reach the park's campground, picnic areas,
and the short trail to the viewpoints and tidepools
around Tongue Point, you go straight at the Striped
Peak Trailhead turnoff and proceed about 0.5 mile,
going through the campground, to the Tongue Point
Picnic and Day-Use Area.

Trail Description

The wide gravel Striped Peak Trail departs from the
northeast corner of the small parking lot ►1 and
travels through a dense second-growth forest of
mixed evergreen and deciduous trees. Salmonberry,
elderberry, stinging nettle, sword fern, and a host
of other plants crowd every inch of the understory.
After about 0.2 mile of gentle downhill, a spur trail
goes left toward the campground, but you turn right

and soon pass a sign informing you that a local Boy Scout troop is responsible for maintaining this trail (thanks, guys!). Here the trail leaves the county park, enters Washington Department of Natural Resources land, and turns to a dirt surface.

The path can sometimes be muddy as it goes gradually up and down in forest and through virtual tunnels of dense shrubbery. Below you on the left, the waters of the Strait of Juan de Fuca gently lap at a rocky shoreline. The trail goes up a couple of very short switchbacks, and it then makes a short but fairly steep descent before passing a nice viewpoint and coming to an unsigned junction ►2 at just more than 0.9 mile.

 Steep

 Viewpoint

The trail that goes straight here is the path that climbs 800 feet over the next 1.6 miles to an outlook atop a ridge east of Striped Peak. This is worthwhile, but you have to share the overlook with people who drove over gravel logging roads to reach the same spot, and the landscape, while good, is not particularly outstanding in comparison to some of the other trail-accessible locations on the Olympic Peninsula.

A shorter and more satisfying option is to go sharply left at the junction. This 0.15-mile trail steeply descends seven short switchbacks, passing a lacy seasonal waterfall near the bottom, to The Cove. ►3 (Really? They couldn't come up with a better name than that?) This little pocket inlet, with its tiny beach and rocky shores, offers excellent tidepooling, very good scenery, and, usually, total solitude. It is the perfect location for a lunch break and some quiet contemplation of nature before you head back to the trailhead. ►4

 Steep

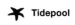 Tidepool

As previously mentioned, be sure to leave plenty of time and energy once you return from your hike to explore the many other fun destinations in Salt Creek County Park. Especially recommended is low-tide exploring of the tidepools around Tongue Point and poking around on lovely Crescent Bay.

Tidepool

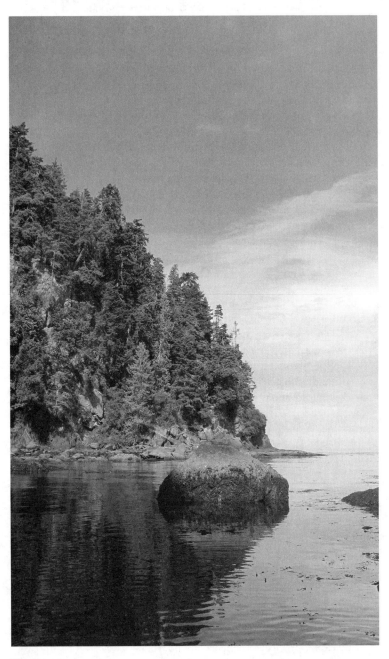

The Cove

Tip: At *really* low tide, you can walk over a rugged rocky area that connects these two locations.

🚶 MILESTONES

▶1   0.0   Striped Peak Trailhead (N48° 09.738' W123° 41.909')
▶2   0.9   Unsigned junction (N48° 09.711' W123° 40.920')
▶3   1.1   The Cove (N48° 09.791' W123° 40.875')
▶4   2.2   Return to trailhead (N48° 09.738' W123° 41.909')

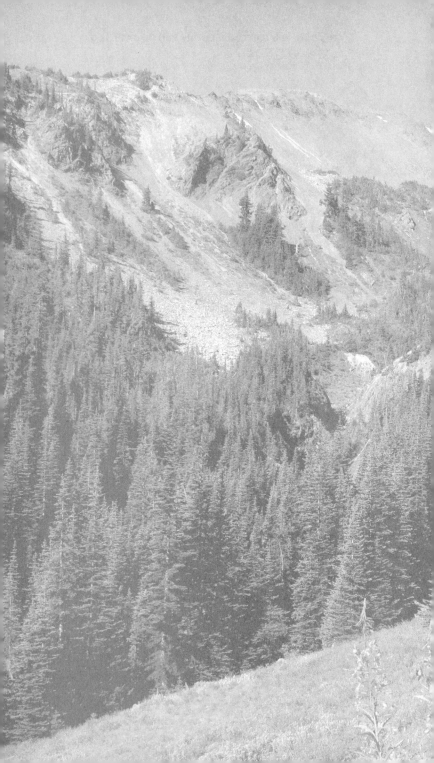

CHAPTER 4

North Central Region: Elwha and Hurricane Ridge Areas

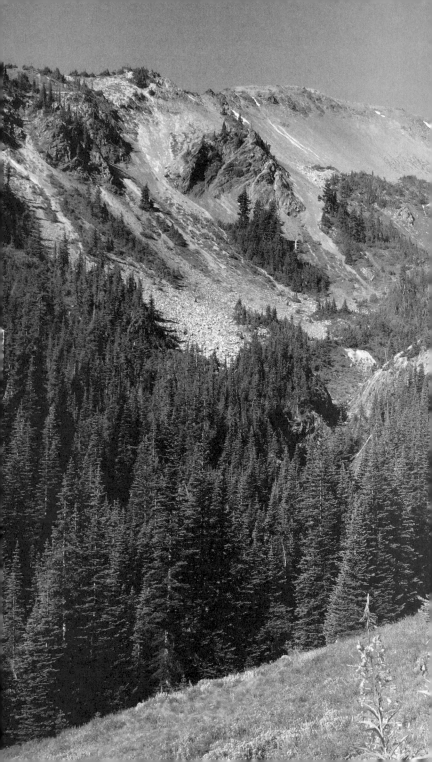

North Central Region: Elwha and Hurricane Ridge Areas

D ue to the close proximity to Port Angeles, the largest city on the Olympic Peninsula, the trails in the North Central region inevitably see a large number of visitors. When you throw in the fact that Hurricane Ridge is the only high-elevation environment in the park accessible by a paved road, then the crowds become even more understandable. But, in fairness, even if the trails here were hidden away in some remote corner of the peninsula, they would still be sought out by the booted masses because they are just so beautiful and fun to hike. The famous views from the meadows atop Hurricane Ridge, so often depicted on postcards or shown in calendars, are unquestionably among the best in the park. The wildflowers are plentiful and extremely colorful, and they fill the mountain air with their wonderful aromas. And the wildlife is both common and friendly, with sightings of deer, marmots, mountain goats, a host of birds, and numerous other critters not just commonplace but virtually guaranteed.

Just to the west of Hurricane Ridge is the Elwha River Valley, a heavily forested low-elevation environment bisected by the longest and perhaps the most enchantingly beautiful river on the peninsula, which is saying something. Fun and relatively easy trails explore the meadows, forests, and canyons of this valley and even visit a handful of old homesteads, evidence that the merits of this region were clear to earlier visitors as well.

Even though the road up to Hurricane Ridge is plowed of snow and kept open all year, the same is not true of the trails, so the hiking season at these high elevations is relatively short. It varies from year to year, but typically the snow has melted enough for summer hiking by late June, and the first snows of winter fall in October. Even in midsummer, however, hikers need to be prepared for the possibility of cold rain and frequent wind. The first

Overleaf and opposite: *Meadow along trail down from Lillian Ridge (Trail 27)*

three times I visited Hurricane Ridge, I was so socked in by clouds, wind, and a cold fog that I couldn't see a thing and assumed all those beautiful postcards were nothing but a cruel joke dreamed up by the local chamber of commerce. But when the skies do clear—and they actually do fairly frequently in the summer, despite my initial bad luck—it is absolutely glorious and the hiking is a joy.

If you are visiting in the off-season, or if the weather gods are throwing another hissy fit, then head for the Elwha River Valley instead. This lower-elevation environment is often open all year, though occasional snow and ice storms may close the access road for periods of time. In addition, when the weather is cold and windy, a hike in the forest is much more comfortable (and safer) than hiking on an open alpine ridge.

Note: The long-awaited removal of the Glines Canyon Dam on the lower Elwha River (to enhance fish habitat) began in late 2011 and is scheduled to last at least through the end of 2014. During the removal process, the Olympic Hot Springs Road and Trail will be closed to all public access. Thus such beautiful and popular trails as those to Appleton Pass, Boulder Lake, and Happy Lake are not currently hikable and have not been included in this edition of this book.

Governing Agency

All the hikes described in this region are administered by Olympic National Park.

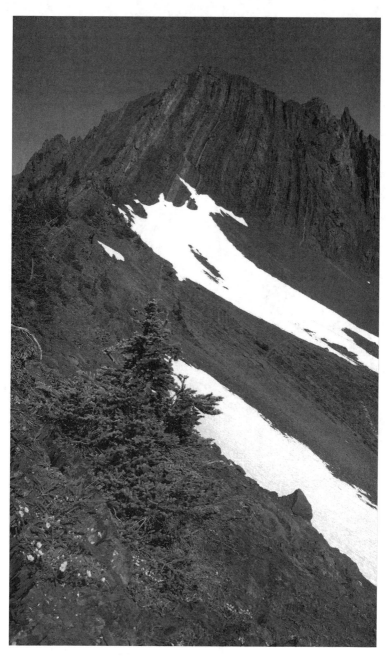

Mount Angeles *from Victor Pass (Trail 23)*

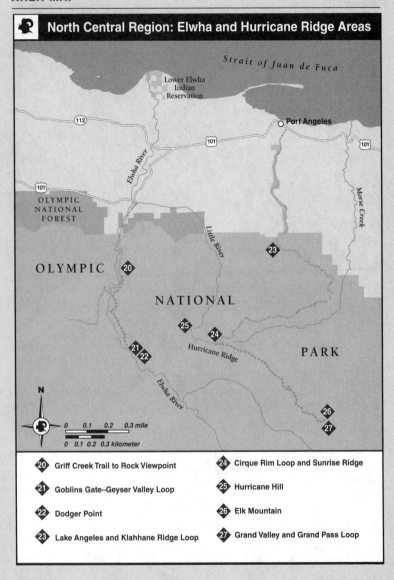

North Central Region: Elwha and Hurricane Ridge Areas

20	Griff Creek Trail to Rock Viewpoint	**24**	Cirque Rim Loop and Sunrise Ridge
21	Goblins Gate–Geyser Valley Loop	**25**	Hurricane Hill
22	Dodger Point	**26**	Elk Mountain
23	Lake Angeles and Klahhane Ridge Loop	**27**	Grand Valley and Grand Pass Loop

TRAIL FEATURES TABLE

North Central Region: Elwha and Hurricane Ridge Areas

TRAIL	DIFFICULTY	LENGTH	TYPE	USES & ACCESS	TERRAIN	FLORA & FAUNA	OTHER
20	4	3.2					
21	3	5.9					
22	5	27.0					
23	4–5	7.4–12.9					
24	1–2	1.1–2.9					
25	2 and 4	3.2–6.4					
26	3	5.0					
27	5	13.9					

USES & ACCESS
- Day Hiking
- Backpacking
- Mountain Biking
- Horses
- Dogs Allowed
- Child-Friendly

TYPE
- Loop
- Semi-loop
- Out-and-back

DIFFICULTY
- 1 2 3 4 5 +
less   more

TERRAIN
- Summit
- Steep
- Lake
- Waterfall
- Tidepool

FLORA & FAUNA
- Old-Growth Forest
- Wildflowers
- Birds
- Wildlife

OTHER
- Viewpoint
- Geologic Interest
- Historic Interest

North Central Region:
Elwha and Hurricane Ridge Areas

TRAIL 20

Day hiking
3.2 miles
Out-and-back
Difficulty: 1 2 3 **4** 5

Griff Creek Trail to Rock Viewpoint . 183

You'll probably huff and puff a lot as you climb this short but tiring little trail, but that extra effort brings commensurate rewards: solitude, plenty of wildlife, rock-garden wildflowers, and a terrific little viewpoint overlooking the wild valley of the Elwha River.

TRAIL 21

Day hiking, back-
packing, horses,
child-friendly
5.9 miles
Semi-loop
Difficulty: 1 2 **3** 4 5

Goblins Gate–Geyser Valley Loop ... 187

The best day hike (or very easy overnight) sampler of the Elwha River Valley, this semi-loop trip visits impressive forests, a couple of lush meadows, and plenty of fine viewpoints beside the beautiful Elwha River. All of which would be more than enough to recommend this hike, but for added interest (actually *lots* of added interest), you will also come across a dramatic rocky gorge and two historic old homesteads, and you will (probably) see some wildlife along the way as well.

TRAIL 22

Backpacking, horses
27.0 miles
Out-and-back
Difficulty: 1 2 3 4 **5**

Dodger Point 193

This long and mostly waterless uphill trail leads to a remote but breathtaking viewpoint from a historic lookout building deep in the heart of the Olympic Mountains. The length of the approach trail ensures that Dodger Point is rarely visited, but were it easier to reach, it would surely be one of the most sought-after viewpoints in the region.

Lake Angeles and
Klahhane Ridge Loop 200

Take your pick: a moderately difficult hike to a
lovely mountain lake or a very challenging but classic loop trip that showcases all of the many charms
of the Hurricane Ridge region, including beautiful
lower-elevation forests, a gorgeous lake with great
camping, high mountain meadows with lots of wildflowers, and a rugged alpine ridge with unbeatable
views. This trip has it all. The full loop, however, is
strictly for well-conditioned and experienced hikers.

TRAIL 23

Day hiking,
backpacking
7.4–12.9 miles
Out-and-back/Loop
Difficulty: 1 2 3 **4 5**

Cirque Rim Loop and
Sunrise Ridge 207

The famous vistas and wildflowers from the
Hurricane Ridge Road are hard to improve upon,
but these short trails manage to pull off that difficult trick. Expect crowds on the paved nature trails
of the Cirque Rim Loop, but you can find surprising solitude by adding a wonderful side trip along
Sunrise Ridge. Given the crowds, it's surprising that
wildlife sightings are an added bonus for most visitors, especially in the morning.

TRAIL 24

Day hiking,
child-friendly
1.1–2.9 miles
Loop/Out-and-back
Difficulty: **1 2** 3 4 5

Hurricane Hill 213

Although one of the busiest trails in the park, this
paved route leads to a stunning high mountain
viewpoint that really should not be missed. Hikers
seeking seclusion, and who are willing to make
a steep side trip, can enjoy equally great views
without all the fellow admirers along a lonesome
subsidiary trail from near the top of Hurricane Hill.
Done together, these two destinations add up to an
unparalleled day of scenic mountain hiking.

TRAIL 25

Day hiking,
child-friendly
3.2–6.4 miles
Out-and-back
Difficulty: 1 **2** 3 4 5

At the western end of aptly named Grand Ridge, Elk Mountain has the highest maintained trails in Olympic National Park and offers views to match. Because the trailhead is already at a high elevation, the hike to this alpine paradise is fairly short and easy and is accessible to anyone willing to make a rather bumpy drive and a steep climb on a narrow and rocky trail.

A popular overnight hike (a reserved permit is recommended) but also accessible to strong day hikers, Grand Valley is a terrific destination featuring a string of sparkling lakes, gorgeous meadows, and generally sublime mountain scenery. The trip starts with a view-packed ramble on an alpine ridge and then plunges more than 1,600 feet into the valley. After a highly recommended side trip to wildly scenic Grand Pass, return on a loop trail through the wildflower-choked meadows of Badger Valley. It's a tough climb back to your car, so allow plenty of time and energy for the return trip.

Griff Creek Trail
to Rock Viewpoint

The best trail-accessible viewpoint of the lower Elwha River Valley is found on the little-traveled Griff Creek Trail, where solitude is virtually assured. It's not as if this trail is hidden or hard to reach; after all, it starts from a good paved road right beside the Elwha Ranger Station. The stiff climb, however, discourages most hikers, who go instead to the better-known paths in Geyser Valley or to Appleton Pass. But don't make that same mistake because Rock Viewpoint at the end of this challenging little hike is worth every tiring step and repays your sweat equity with the best of interest: marvelous views and a blessedly natural return on investment.

Best Time

The trail is usually open April–November, but it's most enjoyable in spring and fall. Avoid hot days because the climb is steep and tiring. The best plan is to try to do the hike in the cool shade of the morning.

Finding the Trail

Drive US 101 about 8 miles west of Port Angeles to a junction at milepost 239.6, where the highway makes a prominent 90-degree turn just east of a bridge over the Elwha River. Turn south on Olympic Hot Springs Road, following signs for the Elwha Valley, and proceed on this paved road for 4.1 miles, entering Olympic National Park and passing a pay station along the way, to the Elwha Ranger Station on the left. Park here.

TRAIL USE
Day hiking

LENGTH
3.2 miles, 2.5 hours

CUMULATIVE ELEVATION
1,470'

DIFFICULTY
- 1 2 3 **4** 5 +

TRAIL TYPE
Out-and-back

SURFACE TYPE
Dirt

CONTOUR MAP
Custom Correct *Elwha Valley*

START & END
N48° 01.002'
W123° 35.415'

FEATURES
Views of the Elwha Valley, solitude

FACILITIES
Restrooms, water, ranger station

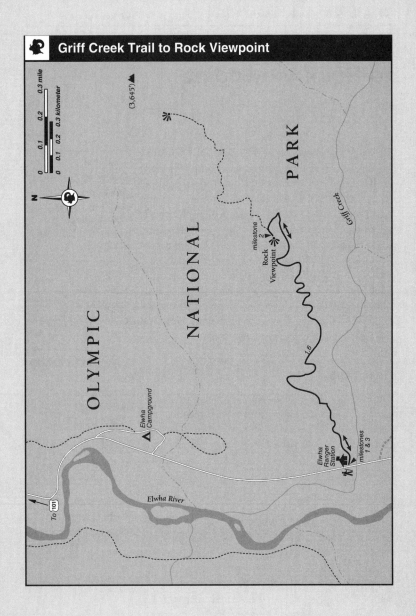

Griff Creek Trail to Rock Viewpoint

0.3 mile
0.2
0.1
0
0.3 kilometer
0.2
0.1
0

N

(3,645')

PARK

milestone
2

Griff Creek

Rock
Viewpoint

NATIONAL

1.6

OLYMPIC

Elwha
Campground

Elwha
Ranger
Station

milestones
1 & 3

To 101

Elwha River

Trail Description

Walk around to the back side of the ranger station building ▶1 and pick up your route at a small sign announcing GRIFF CREEK TRAIL. After leaving the little meadow that holds the ranger station and its assorted buildings, the trail enters a dense and shady forest. You will soon bless that shade because, after a brief warm-up on relatively gentle tread, you then begin a steep and steady climb. The sound of cascading Griff Creek in the canyon on your right is soon left behind, or perhaps it's simply drowned out by all the panting and wheezing. On the plus side, the trail is lonesome, so wildlife sightings are common. Look for deer, black bears, snowshoe hares, and pileated woodpeckers, among other interesting critters. Another bonus is that the forest is unusually attractive, with lots of showy sword ferns on the forest floor. About 20 mostly short and irregularly spaced switchbacks add a bit of variety and keep the uphill grade a bit more reasonable.

At a little more than 1 punishing mile, the forest begins to open up somewhat and include a few Pacific madrone trees, with their distinctive cinnamon-colored bark. Finally, at about 1.5 miles, the prospects for views improve when you cross an open slope below a rocky promontory. Just 0.1 mile and one uphill switchback later takes

Steep

Wildlife

Viewpoint

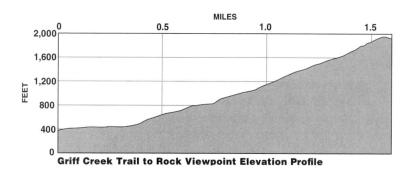
Griff Creek Trail to Rock Viewpoint Elevation Profile

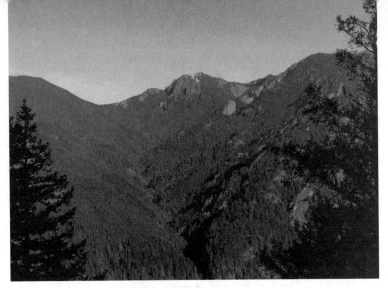

View west *to Happy Lake Ridge from Rock Viewpoint*

you to the signed junction with a 20-yard side trail that goes left to Rock Viewpoint. ▶2

Despite the unimaginative name, this is a dramatic location with superb views up and down the Elwha Valley, across the canyon to Happy Lake Ridge, up the Elwha Canyon to icy Mount Carrie and the Bailey Range, and down to the former site of Glines Canyon Dam and now-drained Lake Mills. In May and June wildflowers add color to the rocky areas around the viewpoint, including such showy favorites as Indian paintbrush, death camas, stonecrop, and Lomatium. Though Griff Creek Trail keeps climbing for another 1.2 miles and passes at least one more good viewpoint along the way, the extra effort is not really worth it because Rock Viewpoint is at least as good as anything farther up the trail. So simply enjoy this spot, and then return to the trailhead. ▶3

Wildflowers

🚶	**MILESTONES**	
▶1	0.0	Take trail from ranger station (N48° 01.002' W123° 35.415')
▶2	1.6	Rock Viewpoint (N48° 01.228' W123° 34.360')
▶3	3.2	Return to trailhead (N48° 01.002' W123° 35.415')

Goblins Gate–Geyser Valley Loop

The Elwha River is one of the longest and largest streams on the Olympic Peninsula and is certainly in the running for the prettiest. Its rushing clear-to-emerald-green waters drain a very scenic canyon flanked by heavily forested ridges. The entire drainage is surrounded by arguably the most sublime mountains in the range and includes some of the most beautiful lower-elevation meadows in the region. The area is also home to a wide assortment of wildlife (elk, bear, and deer) and some fascinating historic log cabins. A very popular and enjoyable trail travels the entire length of this magnificent canyon before climbing over Low Divide and exiting via the North Fork Quinault River Trail to the south. This historic 44-mile trail, which traces the route of the Press Expedition that made the first known crossing of the Olympic Mountains, is a favorite of backpackers. Day hikers can enjoy a superb sampling of this terrain on this pleasant and relatively easy semi-loop trip through Geyser Valley.

Best Time

The trail is often open all year but is reliably hikable from about March to early December. It is most attractive with the abundant greenery and high waters of mid- to late spring. Wildlife viewing is best in winter and early spring. In the summer, try to visit on a weekday because the trail is quite popular. Or visit on a day when the weather is cloudy or rainy.

TRAIL USE
Day hiking, back-packing, horses, child-friendly

LENGTH
5.9 miles, 3 hours

CUMULATIVE ELEVATION
600'

DIFFICULTY
- 1 2 **3** 4 5 +

TRAIL TYPE
Semi-loop

SURFACE TYPE
Dirt

CONTOUR MAP
Custom Correct *Elwha Valley* or Green Trails *Mt Olympus* #134

START & END
N47° 58.075'
W123° 34.950'

FEATURES
Beautiful river, wildlife, peaceful forest, historic cabins

FACILITIES
Restrooms, picnic table, trash can

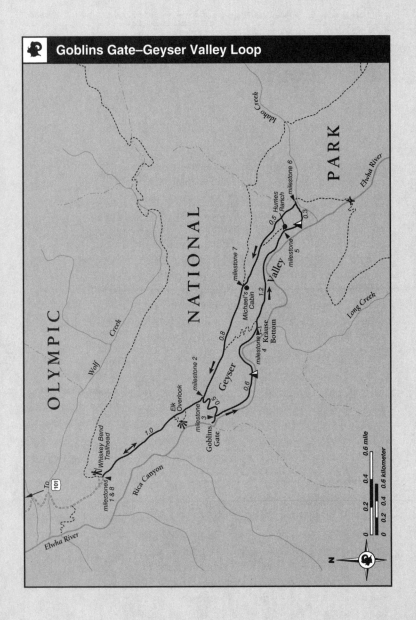

OLYMPIC

NATIONAL

PARK

Idaho Creek

Elwha River

Long Creek

Wolf Creek

Elwha River

Rica Canyon

To 101

milestone 6

0.3

Humes Ranch

0.5

milestone 5

milestone 7

Michael's Cabin

1.2

Geyser Valley

Krause Bottom

milestone 4

0.6

0.8

milestone 2

Elk Overlook

0.5

milestone 3

Goblins Gate

1.0

Whiskey Bend Trailhead

milestones 1 & 8

0.6 mile

0.4

0.2

0.6 kilometer

0.4

0.2

0

N

Finding the Trail

Drive US 101 about 8 miles west of Port Angeles to a junction at milepost 239.5, where the highway makes a prominent 90-degree turn just east of a bridge over the Elwha River. Turn south on Olympic Hot Springs Road, following signs for the Elwha Valley, and proceed on this paved road for 4.1 miles, entering Olympic National Park and passing a pay station along the way, to the Elwha Ranger Station. Continue another 0.2 mile, and then turn left onto Whiskey Bend Road. Drive this narrow gravel road for 4.6 miles to the road-end turnaround and trailhead parking lot.

Trail Description

Two trails leave from this popular trailhead. For this hike, you take the main Elwha Trail, which goes southeast from the end of the road's turn-around loop. ▶1

The wide dirt trail heads up the deep canyon of the Elwha River, staying on the hillside about 450 feet above the cascading water. By Olympic standards, the second-growth forest here is relatively open, allowing for occasional nice views across the canyon to the snow-topped ridge to the west. The trail is remarkably gentle, being either level or with a gradual downhill grade.

At 0.8 mile, a trail marked simply OVERLOOK angles downhill and to the right. After two switchbacks, this moderately graded side trail takes you to Elk Overlook, a rocky promontory with a partial view down to the Elwha River and a meadow on the opposite shore that was once part of the Anderson Ranch homestead. Today, elk are commonly seen in this meadow, but you will need binoculars to get a close look. A very steep return route takes you back up to the Elwha Trail.

 Viewpoint

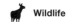 Wildlife

Another gentle 0.2 mile on the main trail takes you to the start of the loop at a signed junction. ▶2 You turn right, following signs to Rica Canyon, and descend seven moderately steep switchbacks to a junction immediately adjacent to the lovely greenish-blue Elwha River. Set aside 10 minutes here for a side trip that goes straight and, in a little under 0.1 mile, takes you to a dramatic rock outcrop directly above Goblins Gate. ▶3 Here, the Elwha River charges through a narrow rock chasm in an impressive display of hydropower. Below the Goblins Gate portal, the river races through the steep confines of virtually inaccessible Rica Canyon.

The main loop trail goes sharply left at the Goblins Gate junction and heads upstream into a relatively flat and gentle section of the Elwha Canyon called Geyser Valley. Although there are no geysers here, there are plenty of big trees, nice views, pretty meadows, and generally pleasant scenery. The circuitous trail provides for easy hiking, as it stays almost level, following a heavily forested bench beside the river. Not quite 0.4 mile from the Goblins Gate turn-off, you pass a 25-yard side path to a very inviting riverside campsite on your right. The next 0.1 mile is a dramatically scenic section where the trail was created by blasting into rock just above the river, offering fine views across the water to the tall ridge to the west. From there, it's back to forest hiking, but this time on a steep little uphill that takes you to a junction with a side trail that goes right to Krause Bottom. ▶4 This short dead-end path curves downhill to a brushy riverside flat.

The main loop trail goes left at the Krause Bottom turnoff and in just 30 yards comes to another junction, this time with a cutoff route that goes left and climbs back up to the main Elwha Trail. You keep right and go up and down in forest for about 0.3 mile before reaching a narrow little meadow. At the upper end of this meadow is a short side trail

Steep

Geologic Interest

Viewpoint

Historic Interest

that goes left to the historic log structure called Humes Ranch. ▶5 An interpretive sign gives the fascinating history of this place and the two brothers, Will and Martin Humes, who built it. A trail goes uphill and to the left here, providing a possible shortcut back to the Elwha Trail.

For the full exploration of Geyser Valley, keep right at the Humes Ranch junction and descend briefly to the large flat known as Humes Meadow. Early in the morning, this is a good place to watch for deer, bears, and elk. There are several excellent and very comfortable campsites here, with a bear wire available near the upper end of the meadow.

 Wildlife

The trail climbs from the meadow for about 0.1 mile to a junction ▶6 a little before you reach Idaho Creek. The trail to the right heads toward Dodger Point. (See Trail 22.) If you have some extra energy, it's worthwhile taking this steep, up-and-down path

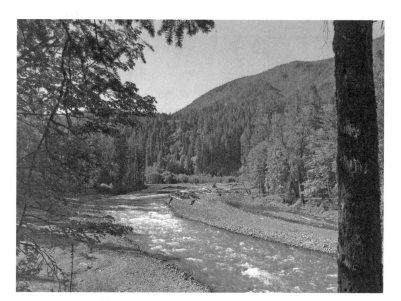

Elwha River *above Goblins Gate*

for about 0.5 mile to the trail bridge across the Elwha River, where you'll enjoy some fine views.

To do the recommended loop, go left at this junction and very gradually ascend the forested hillside above Humes Meadow and the Elwha River. After a little less than 0.3 mile, you come to a junction with the shortcut trail coming up from Humes Ranch. Go straight; just 0.2 mile later, return to the Elwha Trail. Immediately on your left is a tiny pocket meadow and another historic log structure, this one called Michael's Cabin. ►7 The cabin was named for a locally famous hunter known as "Cougar Mike," who made his living by maintaining trails and hunting predators.

Historic Interest 🏠

To return to the trailhead, go straight at the junction, taking the nearly level Elwha Trail as it passes the junction with the Krause Bottom Trail in 0.4 mile and returns to the Rica Canyon junction in another 0.4 mile. Go straight and retrace your route to the trailhead. ►8

🚶 MILESTONES

►1	0.0	Take trail from parking lot (N47° 58.075' W123° 34.950')
►2	1.0	Rica Canyon junction (N47° 57.395' W123° 34.052')
►3	1.5	Goblins Gate (N47° 57.374' W123° 34.513')
►4	2.1	Krause Bottom junction (N47° 57.121' W123° 33.495')
►5	3.3	Humes Ranch (N47° 56.975' W123° 32.824')
►6	3.6	Dodger Point junction (N47° 56.855' W123° 32.458')
►7	4.1	Michael's Cabin (N47° 57.206' W123° 33.240')
►8	5.9	Return to the trailhead (N47° 58.075' W123° 34.950')

Dodger Point

Located near the center of the Olympic Mountains, the old lookout building at Dodger Point is ideally situated to offer an outstanding view of all parts of this magnificent range. And boy does it ever! Just about every significant mountain, glacier, ridge, and canyon is visible from this grandstand, and simply saying, "Wow!" really doesn't cover it. Be prepared to be awed. You should also be prepared, however, to lug a heavy overnight pack on a long uphill trail, which probably explains why only a small number of hikers ever get to appreciate this wonderful view. This is fine for solitude lovers, of course, who enjoy the view even more knowing that they have it all to themselves.

Note: The Long Ridge Trail to Dodger Point is one of the few trails in Olympic National Park where finding water can be a problem. By late summer, there may be no accessible trailside water between Idaho Creek and the small ponds in Dodger Basin, a distance of 10.4 tough, uphill miles. Carry plenty.

Best Time

The trail to Dodger Point is usually open July–October. Clear weather is needed to fully appreciate the views.

Finding the Trail

Drive US 101 about 8 miles west of Port Angeles to a junction at milepost 239.5, where the highway makes a prominent 90-degree turn just east of a bridge over the Elwha River. Turn south on

TRAIL USE
Backpacking, horses
LENGTH
27.0 miles, 2–3 days
**CUMULATIVE
ELEVATION**
5,300'
DIFFICULTY
- 1 2 3 4 **5** +
TRAIL TYPE
Out-and-back
SURFACE TYPE
Dirt
CONTOUR MAP
Custom Correct *Elwha
Valley*
START & END
N47° 58.075'
W123° 34.950'

FEATURES
Mountain viewpoint,
historic lookout build-
ing, solitude, long ridge
walk

FACILITIES
Restrooms, picnic
table, trash can

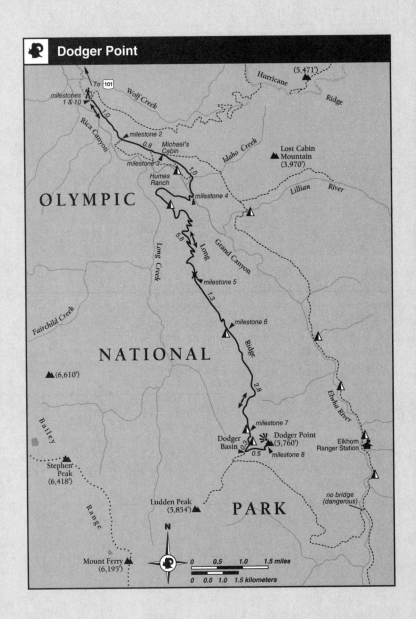

To [101]

milestones
1 & 10

Wolf Creek

Rica Canyon

Hurricane

(5,471')

Ridge

1.0

milestone 2

0.8

Michael's
Cabin

milestone 3

Idaho Creek

Lost Cabin
Mountain
(3,970')

1.0

Humes
Ranch

milestone 4

Lillian

River

OLYMPIC

5.8

Long

Grand Canyon

Long Creek

milestone 5

1.3

Fairchild Creek

milestone 6

NATIONAL

Ridge

(6,610')

2.8

Elwha River

milestone 7

Dodger
Basin

0.3

Dodger Point
(5,760')

Elkhorn
Ranger Station

Stephen
Peak
(6,418')

0.5

milestone 8

Bailey

Ludden Peak
(5,854')

PARK

no bridge
(dangerous)

Range

N

Mount Ferry
(6,195')

0   0.5   1.0   1.5 miles

0   0.5   1.0   1.5 kilometers

Olympic Hot Springs Road, following signs for the Elwha Valley, and proceed on this paved road for 4.1 miles, entering Olympic National Park and passing a pay station along the way, to the Elwha Ranger Station. Continue another 0.2 mile, and then turn left onto Whiskey Bend Road. Drive this narrow gravel road for 4.6 miles to the road-end turnaround and trailhead parking lot.

Trail Description

The trailhead ►1 is located at the southeast end of the parking turnaround beside a large signboard. Follow the wide, smooth, and heavily used Elwha Trail as it goes gently up and down across a densely forested hillside. You can hear the Elwha River as it rushes through Rica Canyon far below you on the right, and you will see glimpses of a tall, heavily forested ridge across the Elwha Valley to the west. At 0.8 mile, you go straight where a signed side trail drops to the right toward Elk Overlook, and then at 1 mile come to the junction with the Rica Canyon Trail. ►2 This trail offers a somewhat more scenic but longer alternate route. See Trail 21 for details.

For the shorter and more direct route, go straight at the junction, still on the Elwha Trail, which remains very gentle and in generally viewless

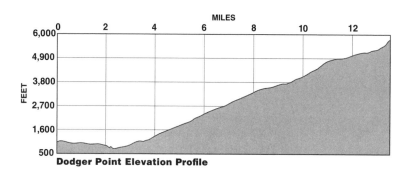

Dodger Point Elevation Profile

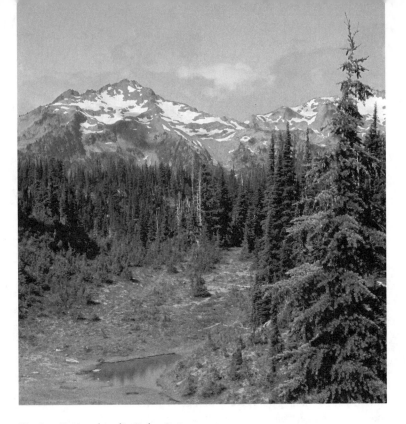

Stephen Peak *and pond in Dodger Basin*

Historic Interest

forest. You go straight again where a trail angles down to the right toward Krause Bottom and then come to another junction beside the small meadow holding the historic old log structure of Michael's Cabin. ▶3

You leave the Elwha Trail at this junction and bear right, following signs to Dodger Point and Humes Meadow. Just 0.2 mile later is another trail fork. If you are making it a short first day, you'll want to go right here toward the campsites near Humes Ranch. The main route to Dodger Point, however, keeps left and goes gently downhill for 0.3 mile to a junction just before you reach splashing Idaho Creek. The return trail up from the campsites at Humes Ranch meets your trail here. Go straight and cross small Idaho Creek shortly after this junction. *Note:* This creek is the last reliable and easily accessible water source until you reach the two small ponds in Dodger Basin, fully 10.4 miles of tough uphill away. Be sure to fill your water bottles here.

After crossing Idaho Creek, the trail does some steep little ups and downs on a newer section of tread that goes around a large washout. This takes you to a tall wood-and-metal bridge suspended high over the Elwha River. ▶4

 Steep

Once across the bridge, you start the long, tiring uphill to Dodger Point. The trail is exceptionally well graded, so except for the last 0.5 mile it is never steep. Even so, you will gain a full 4,900 feet over the next 10.7 miles, so settle in for a *long* haul. The first two of what will be many switchbacks begin less than 0.1 mile past the bridge. These first two zigzags are followed by an extended traverse of about 1 mile, leading to the rounded end of well-named Long Ridge. Here the path curves to the left and travels near the top of the wide ridge for about 0.4 mile to a nice (but dry) campsite.

The trail now temporarily switches to the west side of the forested ridge, continuing its steady but gradual ascent to the next switchback, which takes you back over the ridge to the east side of the divide. By Olympic standards, the forest here is relatively open, allowing partial views to the northeast of Hurricane Ridge as you climb. That climb begins to feel unending as you switchback another 15 times up the east side of the ridge, though rarely straying too far from the top of the divide. Eventually, you reach a little saddle and, immediately beyond, come to a sign at the 3,500-foot point ▶5 stating that NO OPEN FIRES ALLOWED ABOVE THIS POINT—STOVES ONLY.

 Viewpoint

For the next few miles, the trail remains faithful to the west side of Long Ridge as it makes a gradual uphill traverse. The forests now change to higher-elevation species, with fewer Douglas-firs and western hemlocks and more mountain hemlocks and subalpine firs. About 1 mile from the saddle, you pass two tiny springs where you *might* be able to obtain water (don't count on it), and then make two quick switchbacks and pass a small campsite ▶6 beside another unreliable trickle. The forest in this area is a bit more open, allowing you partial and tantalizing views of rugged Stephen Peak and the icy Bailey Range to the west.

As you near the top of your long ascent, you gradually break out of the trees and enter Dodger Basin, which is covered with only partial forest and scattered heather meadows that offer more unobstructed views. In the middle of this pretty basin, you pass above a pair of very shallow and meadow-rimmed ponds ▶7 that offer your first reliable water since Idaho Creek.

There are mediocre campsites near these ponds, but for a better and more hidden campsite, keep hiking another 0.1 mile to a rocky basin beneath Dodger Point, where there is a seasonal creek. Because the creek is usually dry where it crosses the trail, this doesn't look too promising for a campsite. If you follow an unsigned but obvious boot trail that goes to the left a few yards after you cross the dry creek, however, things quickly improve. After about 60 yards, this side trail takes you to a small spring and trickle of water that is almost always reliable. On a partly forested bench just above this trickle is an excellent campsite, with good views. This is also a great place to sit and watch the sunset in the evening.

To reach Dodger Point, follow the main trail another 0.2 mile past the creek crossing to a junction on a little ridge. The trail to the right goes west toward Ludden Peak. To reach your goal, however, turn left and climb, moderately steeply at times, up the little ridge. After 0.5 mile, you reach the summit of Dodger Point ▶8 and its small

Viewpoint

Lake

Steep

Summit

Historic Interest

wooden lookout building, which is usually locked and closed to the public.

From this fine grandstand, you can see a large percentage of the Olympic Mountains. Hikers familiar with the range will be able to identify dozens of features, including Hurricane Hill, Hurricane Ridge, and Mount Angeles to the north; Lillian Ridge and McCartney Peak to the east; the deep canyon of the Elwha River and its tributaries; Mounts Wilder and Dana to the south; and, best of all, Mount Ferry, Mount Olympus, and the Bailey Range to the west. You could spend hours here taking it all in before reluctantly heading down to your camp and then making the long hike back to the trailhead ▶9 the way you came.

 Viewpoint

	🚶 MILESTONES	
▶1	0.0	Trailhead (N47° 58.075' W123° 34.950')
▶2	1.0	Rica Canyon junction (N47° 57.395' W123° 34.052')
▶3	1.8	Michael's Cabin junction (N47° 57.206' W123° 33.240')
▶4	2.8	Elwha River Bridge (N47° 56.507' W123° 32.494')
▶5	8.6	Sign at 3,500' (N47° 55.169' W123° 32.401')
▶6	9.9	Small campsite (N47° 54.280' W123° 31.871')
▶7	12.7	Ponds in Dodger Basin (N47° 52.553' W123° 30.975')
▶8	13.5	Dodger Point (N47° 52.449' W123° 30.594')
▶9	27.0	Return to trailhead (N47° 58.075' W123° 34.950')

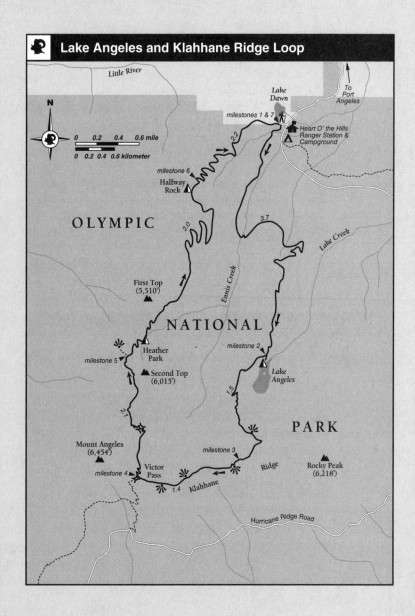

Lake Angeles and Klahhane Ridge Loop

Little River

Lake Dawn

To Port Angeles

milestones 1 & 7

2.2

Heart O' the Hills
Ranger Station &
Campground

N

0   0.2   0.4   0.6 mile

0   0.2   0.4   0.6 kilometer

milestone 6

Halfway
Rock

OLYMPIC

2.0

3.7

Lake Creek

Ennis Creek

First Top
(5,510')

NATIONAL

milestone 5

Heather
Park

milestone 2

Lake
Angeles

Second Top
(6,015')

1.5

PARK

2.1

Mount Angeles
(6,454')

milestone 4

Victor
Pass

milestone 3

Ridge

Rocky Peak
(6,218')

1.4   Klahhane

Hurricane Ridge Road

Lake Angeles and Klahhane Ridge Loop

Depending on your mood and abilities, this trip can be either a moderately difficult hike to a lovely mountain lake or a challenging but classic loop trip that showcases all of the many charms of the Hurricane Ridge region. Starting in a low-elevation forest, the trail makes a pleasant climb to large and very attractive Lake Angeles. You could camp or simply turn around here, well satisfied with your efforts. For the best scenery, however, trudge your way up (*way* up) to a dramatic alpine ridge with outstanding views. After a couple of tremendously scenic miles along this rugged ridge, you loop back along a rough trail to your starting point. The full loop is worth every one of the many calories required to do it, but it is only for well-conditioned and experienced hikers.

Best Time

The lower section to Lake Angeles is typically hikable in early June. The full loop is usually open mid-July–October. Wait for a clear day to appreciate the fine views from Klahhane Ridge and be sure to get an early start.

Finding the Trail

From US 101 in downtown Port Angeles, turn south on Race Street, following large signs pointing to Hurricane Ridge and Olympic National Park Visitor Center. This road eventually leaves town, becomes Mount Angeles Road, and passes the Olympic National Park Visitor Center and Wilderness Information Center on the right. At 1.2 miles

TRAIL USE
Day hiking, backpacking

LENGTH
7.4 miles to Lake Angeles, 4 hours (or overnight); 12.9 miles for the loop, 8 hours

CUMULATIVE ELEVATION
2,400' to Lake Angeles; 4,900' for the loop

DIFFICULTY
- 1 2 3 **4 5** +

TRAIL TYPE
Out-and-back or loop

SURFACE TYPE
Dirt

CONTOUR MAP
Custom Correct *Hurricane Ridge*

START & END
N48° 02.325'
W123° 25.898'

FEATURES
Pretty mountain lake, scenic alpine ridge

FACILITIES
None (but restrooms, picnic tables, a campground, and a ranger station are nearby).

201

from US 101 (or 0.1 mile past the visitor center), you bear right at a prominent fork and then continue another 4.3 miles to a road junction immediately before the park's entrance station and pay booth. Turn right here and proceed 0.2 mile to the Lake Angeles Trailhead.

Trail Description

Old-Growth Forest

The wide Lake Angeles Trail begins from the south side of the parking lot ▶1 in a dense and quite beautiful forest of big Douglas-firs, western hemlocks, and western red cedars. The shade these trees provide is nearly complete, which is a good thing because the trail starts right off by going uphill. You'll be doing a lot of that, so settle in and begin climbing. At first the pace is gradual, but it won't stay that way. At 0.1 mile, you take a bridge over a small creek and then ascend a ridgeline, always in viewless but attractive forest. After rounding the little ridge, the trail makes a moderately graded but unrelenting ascent of the canyon of Ennis Creek. For the most part, you stay on the forested hillside just west of the stream, so you'll rarely see the water, but you can always hear it tumbling along beside you.

You take a log bridge over Ennis Creek at about 1.3 miles and then leave its cheerful waters as you

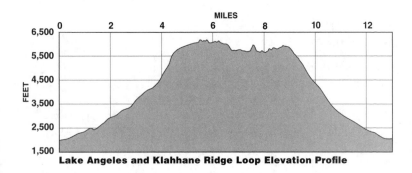

Lake Angeles and Klahhane Ridge Loop Elevation Profile

wind your way up through a small area of heavy blowdown. The trail then climbs around a wide ridge. The uphill continues unabated as you make a series of switchbacks up the ridge, with the trail eventually settling on the east side of the rounded divide. At 3.6 miles, the trail abruptly levels off by a tiny meadow and soon takes you to a signed junction. To see Lake Angeles, ▶2 bear left and about 150 yards later reach a bear box and several good campsites near the lake.

 Lake

Lake Angeles is quite beautiful, surrounded on three sides by towering rock walls and with a pretty little island in the middle. Not surprisingly, these features make the lake a well-visited destination. The trail this far is usually open by June, making the lake a particularly excellent hiking goal in early summer.

If it is later in the summer, however, and you are a strong hiker with plenty of time and energy, then the fun (and the work) is far from over. To make the long and rugged, but highly rewarding, loop, return to the junction just north of Lake Angeles and turn onto the trail for Klahhane Ridge. This trail climbs steeply, much more steeply than the route to Lake Angeles, rapidly taking you into a more open and higher-elevation forest dominated by Alaska yellow cedars and first Pacific silver then subalpine firs. The small openings offer good looks down to the waters of Lake Angeles and across to rugged Rocky Peak.

 Steep

At about 0.4 mile from the lake, you reach a narrow ridge topped with rock-garden wildflowers and impressive rocky pinnacles. From here, you make a brief downhill, switching to the west side of the ridge before resuming your steep uphill grind (don't say I didn't warn you). Before long, you encounter the first pink mountain heather, always a welcome sign that the alpine zone isn't far away and most of the climbing is over. A switchback takes you back over to the east side of the ridge and then 0.3 mile

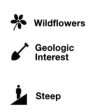
Wildflowers

Geologic Interest

Steep

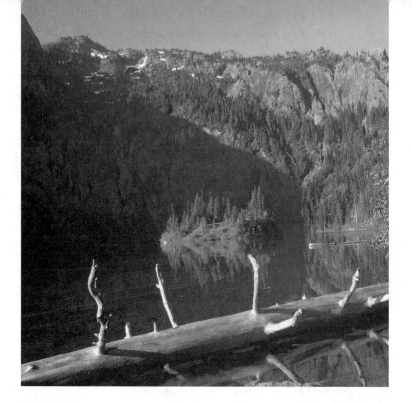

Lake Angeles

of particularly steep climbing before things ease off a bit and you ascend through open subalpine parklands and rocky areas with great views down to Lake Angeles and north to Vancouver Island. You finally top out on Klahhane Ridge, ▶3 pleased in both the scenery and the knowledge that most (though not all) of the hard work is over. Also delightful are the new views to the south and southwest of Mount Olympus, the Bailey Range, and a large portion of the wild Olympic Mountains.

Viewpoint

Steep

The trail turns west along the narrow and rocky ridge, steeply gaining and losing elevation as dictated by the extremely rugged terrain. For a landmark, the prominent peak to the west with the wildly tilted layers of dark rock is Mount Angeles. To the left and more than 1,000 feet below you is Hurricane Ridge Road. The ridge on which you are hiking is a continuing series of rock formations brightened by pretty little clusters of alpine wildflowers, such as lupine, owl's clover, forget-me-not, phlox, Lomatium, Cusick's speedwell, alpine buttercup, yarrow, lousewort, both pink and white mountain heather, and many others. The wildly scenic ridge walk ends at a junction in a saddle just east of the cliffs of Mount Angeles called Victor Pass. ▶4

Geologic Interest

Wildflowers

The main trail goes left here on its way to Hurricane Ridge. For this loop, you turn right on Heather Park Trail and descend a series of four switchbacks toward a rocky basin on the north side of Klahhane Ridge. *Warning:* Be careful of your footing here, and over the next couple of miles, because the trail is often steep, narrow, and covered with loose rocks and pebbles.

Steep

Before reaching the bottom of the basin, the trail cuts to the left and traverses the steep slopes below Mount Angeles and a ridge that goes north from that peak. After skirting some cliffs, the trail climbs a chute of loose rock in a dozen short but steep switchbacks to the top of the ridge, where there are fine views to the west and northwest of the Strait of Juan de Fuca, Hurricane Hill, Unicorn Peak, and many other landmarks.

Viewpoint

The top of the ridge here is much too rugged for a trail, so you are now forced to switchback steeply down the west side of the divide, going around and beneath dark gray and red cliffs and hulking rock formations and pinnacles. After the initial descent, the trail turns north and makes a quite rugged up-and-down traverse of the strangely contorted west side of the ridge. This tiring section ends with a steep little uphill to a small, relatively flat little meadow. ▶5 An unsigned but easy-to-follow spur trail goes left here to a fine viewpoint atop a nearby knoll.

Geologic Interest

Steep

The trail is better constructed and offers easier hiking from here on, as four well-graded downhill switchbacks take you 0.4 mile to an

Old-Growth Forest

inviting designated camping area called Heather Park beside a small but permanent creek. Six more switchbacks lead you down through sloping meadows, and then a long downhill traverse takes you into increasingly dense mid- and lower-elevation forests. The downhill is broken up by scattered switchbacks, and the grade is always reasonable on your tired knees and toes. You pass a good but dry campsite (the former site of a trail shelter) just before coming to Halfway Rock, ▶6 a viewless and nondescript large rock at a switchback. The trail now descends at least 14 more irregularly spaced switchbacks through uneventful but enjoyable forest for 2.2 miles to the trailhead parking lot. ▶7

🚶 MILESTONES

▶1   0.0   Trailhead (N48° 02.325' W123° 25.898')

▶2   3.7   Lake Angeles (N48° 00.516' W123° 26.002')

▶3   5.2   Top of Klahhane Ridge (N47° 59.751' W123° 26.211')

▶4   6.6   Victor Pass junction (N47° 59.604' W123° 27.564')

▶5   8.7   Meadow above Heather Park (N48° 00.557' W123° 27.677')

▶6   10.7   Halfway Rock (N48° 01.912' W123° 26.805')

▶7   12.9   Return to trailhead (N48° 02.325' W123° 25.898')

Cirque Rim Loop and Sunrise Ridge

Some of the best views in Olympic National Park, and certainly its most famous ones, can be had from just off the road at the top of Hurricane Ridge. Millions of people flock here to take in the scene. For those who want to stretch their legs a bit, a fine assortment of fairly easy trails explore the ridgetop's gorgeous meadows and lead to arguably even better viewpoints than those from the road. Be sure to visit when the weather is clear, not only to take in the views, but also so you don't have to deal with walking in the potentially dangerous high winds, rain, or even snow that can hit these high elevations at any time of year.

Best Time

The trails here are usually open (though with some snow patches) from mid- to late June through October. The flowers peak in the latter part of July. A clear day is required to really soak in the outstanding views. Early mornings offer the best photographs, are less crowded, and usually allow you to see more wildlife.

Finding the Trail

From US 101 in downtown Port Angeles, turn south on Race Street, following large signs pointing to Hurricane Ridge and Olympic National Park Visitor Center. This road eventually leaves town, becomes Mount Angeles Road, and passes the Olympic National Park Visitor Center and Wilderness Information Center on the right. At 1.2 miles from US 101 (or 0.1 mile past the visitor center), you bear

TRAIL USE
Day hiking,
child-friendly

LENGTH
1.1 miles for Cirque
Rim Loop, 1 hour; 2.9
miles with Sunrise
Ridge side trip, 2 hours

**CUMULATIVE
ELEVATION**
320' for Cirque Rim
Loop; 800' with Sunrise
Ridge side trip

DIFFICULTY
- **1 2** 3 4 5 +

TRAIL TYPE
Loop or out-and-back

SURFACE TYPE
Paved, gravel, dirt

CONTOUR MAP
Custom Correct
Hurricane Ridge

START & END
N47° 58.201'
W123° 29.703'

FEATURES
Mountain views,
abundant wildflowers,
wildlife viewing, alpine
meadows

FACILITIES
Restrooms, picnic
tables, visitor center

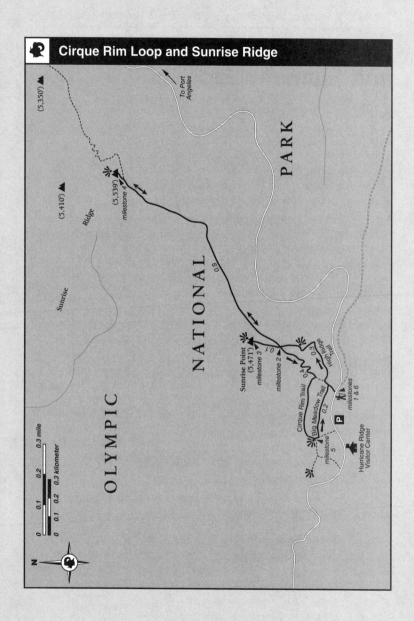

Cirque Rim Loop and Sunrise Ridge

OLYMPIC

NATIONAL

PARK

(5,350')▲

(5,410')▲

Sunrise Ridge

(5,539')▲
milestone 4

To Port Angeles

0.9

Sunrise Point
(5,471')
milestone 3

milestone 2

0.1

High Ridge Trail

0.3

0.4

Cirque Rim Trail

Big Meadow Trail

0.2

milestones 1 & 6

P

milestone 5

Hurricane Ridge Visitor Center

N

0   0.1   0.2   0.3 mile
0   0.1   0.2   0.3 kilometer

right at a prominent fork and then continue another 4.3 miles to the park's entrance station and pay booth. From here, climb the winding and increasingly scenic road for 12.5 miles to the large, but often full, parking lot at the top of Hurricane Ridge. The Hurricane Ridge Visitor Center is visible just ahead on the left.

Trail Description

Any of several excellent loops and walks are possible on the network of nature trails and longer paths radiating out from the Hurricane Ridge parking lot. The recommended itinerary is to start at the trailhead on the north side of the road, across from the east end of the parking lot. ▶1

The paved Cirque Rim Trail goes up a hillside covered with wildflowers and waving subalpine grasses. Signs here admonish visitors to *please* stay on the trail to avoid damaging the very delicate high-elevation plant life. They also demand that hikers not feed the deer, chipmunks, and sometimes mountain goats, which always seem to be around looking cute and photogenic. For the most part, it seems that visitors are heeding this advice because, despite the crowds, the meadows look to be in remarkably good condition, and the animals generally aren't habituated to human handouts. Let's try to keep it that way!

 Wildlife

After only 20 yards, you keep straight where the paved Big Meadow Trail goes left (the recommended return route). Just 30 yards later, you go right on High Ridge Trail. This initially paved trail ascends steadily amid a mix of lovely subalpine meadows and stands of wind-whipped subalpine firs. In mid- to late July, the meadows are filled with colorful wildflowers, and signs help you to identify the many varieties. Some of the more common species include pink mountain heather, broadleaf lupine, scalloped

 Wildflowers

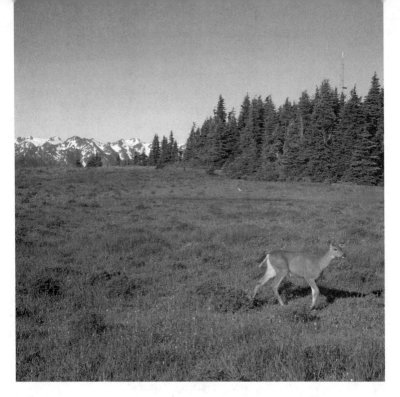

Deer *along Big Meadow Trail on Hurricane Ridge*

Viewpoint

onion, Martindale's Lomatium, American bistort, and Jacob's ladder. And the views are absolutely world-class! Especially outstanding are those to the southwest of the snowy ridges and peaks around Mount Olympus. On a clear day, you'll spend lots of time snapping photographs.

The path soon turns to gravel, shortly before reaching a fine viewpoint with a bench where you can rest. The trail then continues up the little ridge, offering postcard-perfect views down to the visitor center and the mountains beyond as it makes a few short switchbacks to the top of a rocky point at about 0.25 mile. From here, you drop briefly to a saddle and a four-way junction. ▶2

There are no bad options from this junction, and if you have the time and energy, the recommended itinerary is to explore every direction. The shortest alternative, and the best return route, is to turn left and begin hiking downhill back to your car. You'll kick yourself, however, if you don't at least throw in the short ramble to the top of Sunrise Point, the high point right in front of you. So go straight and climb for a little more than 100 yards to the top of the pyramid-shaped summit of Sunrise Point. ▶3 The terrific views from here include not only those to Hurricane Ridge and Mount Olympus, but also excellent vistas to the north of the Strait of Juan de Fuca, Port Angeles, and Canada's Vancouver Island. Sit back and enjoy it all before returning to the four-way junction.

 Summit

Viewpoint

For a short walk, turn right and head back to the trailhead. For those with more time and who want to get away from most of the crowds, however, a longer side trip is possible that is well worth the effort.

To do the side trip, you go sharply left (northeast) at the four-way junction and walk downhill across a meadow-covered hillside. The distinctive peak directly in front of you is Mount Angeles, but there is plenty more to see in all directions. Well below you and on the right is the Hurricane Ridge Road, which you are paralleling. After the hillside traverse ends, the up-and-down trail remains generally on or near the top of the very scenic ridge. At about 0.9 mile from the four-way junction, you reach an unsigned but obvious junction with a 50-yard spur trail that goes left to the top of a high point on Sunrise Ridge. ▶4 This spot offers outstanding 360-degree views including nearby Mount Angeles, back along Sunrise Ridge to Mount Olympus, and of the many peaks, ridges, and forested canyons all around. Because the continuation of the trail makes a significant downhill from here, this knoll is the logical turn-around point for the side trip.

 Summit

 Viewpoint

After returning to the four-way junction, you go right (southwest) on the continuation of High Ridge Trail. This path starts by crossing the northwest side of a little ridge and then makes four quick downhill switchbacks to a reunion with the paved Cirque Rim Trail. Again, you can go left and in no time reach the trailhead. But an extremely easy loop explores more of this scenic terrain, so the recommended course is to turn right and follow the paved trail along a rounded ridgetop with lots of wildflowers, wind-whipped trees, interpretive signs, and, of course, panoramic views.

Viewpoint At the next junction in just 0.2 mile is a developed viewpoint ▶5 lined with a stone wall and including signs pointing out the highlights of the view. Featured in this scene is Hurricane Hill to the northwest (see Trail 25) and evidence of the 2003 Griff Fire to the north–northwest around the pinnacles of Unicorn Horn and Griff Peak.

To return to your car, go left (south) at this viewpoint and left again just 10 yards later on the paved Big Meadow Trail. After 0.15 mile, this well-named and view-filled path takes you back to the junction with Cirque Rim Trail just above the trailhead. ▶6 Turn right and you're there.

🚶	MILESTONES	
▶1	0.0	Trailhead at east end of parking lot (N47° 58.201' W123° 29.703')
▶2	0.3	Four-way junction in saddle (N47° 58.346' W123° 29.512')
▶3	0.4	Sunrise Point (N47° 58.448' W123° 29.463')
▶4	1.4	High point on Sunrise Ridge (N47° 58.845' W123° 28.768')
▶5	2.7	Developed viewpoint (N47° 58.258' W123° 29.888')
▶6	2.9	Return to trailhead (N47° 58.201' W123° 29.703')

Hurricane Hill

You certainly won't be lonesome on this heavily used trail, but the crowds are there for a good reason: an easily accessible trail to a mountain overlook with few equals in the park. The solitude-seeking hiker, however, should not avoid this path because a steep but amazingly quiet side trail departs from near the summit of Hurricane Hill and takes you to a lonesome meadow viewpoint on the ridge to the west. Here, the vistas are just as grand as those from the busy main objective, but even on a nice summer weekend, you'll probably have them all to yourself.

Best Time

The trail to Hurricane Hill is open all year and is actually a popular snowshoe destination in the winter. The path is typically open for summer hiking from mid-June through October. The side trip usually has snow until at least early July. Wait for a clear day to appreciate the views.

Finding the Trail

From US 101 in downtown Port Angeles, turn south on Race Street, following large signs pointing to Hurricane Ridge and Olympic National Park Visitor Center. This road eventually leaves town, becomes Mount Angeles Road, and passes the Olympic National Park Visitor Center and Wilderness Information Center on the right. At 1.2 miles from US 101 (or 0.1 mile past the visitor center), you bear right at a prominent fork and then continue another 4.3 miles to the park's entrance station and pay booth. From here,

TRAIL USE
Day hiking,
child-friendly

LENGTH
3.2 miles to Hurricane
Hill, 1.5–2 hours; 6.4
miles with side trip, 3
hours

**CUMULATIVE
ELEVATION**
700' to Hurricane Hill;
1,700' with side trip

DIFFICULTY
- 1 **2** 3 **4** 5 +

TRAIL TYPE
Out-and-back

SURFACE TYPE
Paved, dirt

CONTOUR MAP
Custom Correct
Hurricane Ridge

START & END
N47° 58.597'
W123° 31.069'

FEATURES
Mountain views,
wildflowers, Olympic
marmots

FACILITIES
None

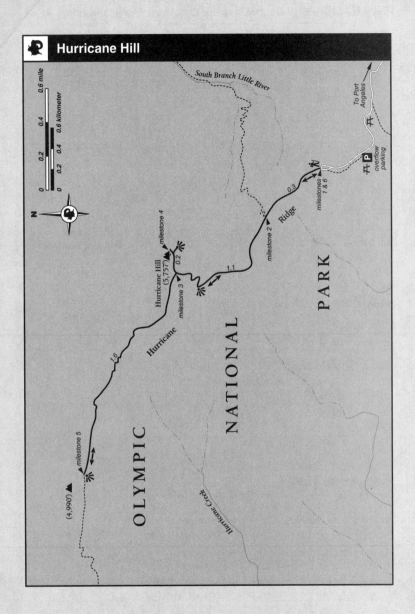

Hurricane Hill

South Branch Little River

To Port Angeles

overflow parking

milestones 1 & 6

0.3

milestone 2

Ridge

2

milestone 4

Hurricane Hill
(5,757')

0.2

1.1

milestone 3

Hurricane

1.6

milestone 5

(4,990')

Hurricane Creek

OLYMPIC   NATIONAL   PARK

N

0   0.2   0.4   0.6 mile
0   0.2   0.4   0.6 kilometer

climb the winding and increasingly scenic road for 12.8 miles to the Hurricane Ridge Visitor Center. At the end of the roadside parking lot here, the road narrows and continues another 1.3 miles to the road-end parking lot for Hurricane Hill. If this lot is full, overflow parking (with a connector trail) is about 0.25 mile back down the road.

Trail Description

The trail begins beside a large signboard at the northwest end of the parking lot. ►1 The path is extremely popular, so the National Park Service has paved the trail to prevent erosion. Help the NPS out by staying on the paved surface and not trampling the delicate plants that cling to life in this high-elevation environment. The route travels through open forests and wildflower-covered meadows, the latter offering great views, especially to the south of such snowy peaks as Mount Carrie, Stephen Peak, and the Bailey Range.

The trail remains almost level for the first 0.3 mile to a ridgetop saddle with an easy-to-miss junction with the Little River Trail. ►2 From here, your route goes straight and climbs a mostly open, south-facing hillside. With the foreground wildflowers, the very deep and heavily forested canyon of the Elwha

 Viewpoint

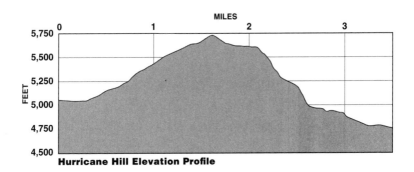

Hurricane Hill Elevation Profile

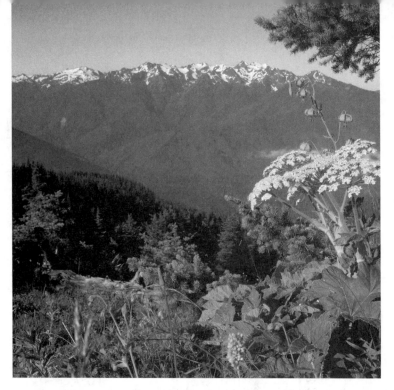

Flowers *and view south from Hurricane Hill Trail*

River and its tributaries, and a skyline filled with snowy and jagged peaks, it is hard to imagine views getting much better than this.

After a short interlude in forest, the trail breaks out into another glorious meadow, this one hosting a particular abundance of American bistort. This flower, with its puff ball top of tiny white blossoms, looks sort of like an oversize cotton swab. Another common resident in this area is the Olympic marmot. This absolutely cute-as-a-button fur ball is about the size of an overweight house cat and offers up high-pitched whistles at passing hikers. Following four moderately long switchbacks in this fine meadow, you come to a junction. ▶3 The dirt trail to the left is a highly recommended side trip, especially if you prefer to enjoy your views with greater solitude.

Before making the side trip, however, you'll want to first visit the top of Hurricane Hill. So keep

Wildflowers

Wildlife

straight at the junction and continue climbing for another 0.2 mile to the end of the paved trail a bit below the actual summit of Hurricane Hill. ▶4 Signs point out the peaks and other major landmarks visible from this terrific grandstand. In addition, short side trails radiate out to other viewing locations, including up to the actual summit of the peak. As always, *please* stay on the maintained trails rather than wandering off across the meadows. With just a few steps, you could destroy years of growth by the tough little plants that struggle to survive here.

 Summit

 Viewpoint

After soaking in the views from the top, go back 0.2 mile to the junction mentioned previously. If you are tired, pressed for time, or have already seen enough, then go back down the paved trail to the parking lot. Hikers looking for more exercise or a less crowded viewpoint, however, should go right (west) following signs to Elwha Trail.

This narrow dirt route follows a scenic ridgeline to the west. The path goes quite steeply downhill at times, losing more than 700 feet in less than a mile: elevation you will have to regain on the return route. You finally level off in meadows on the south side of the ridge and happily ramble along through this scenic landscape for another 0.5 mile or so. Wildflowers, especially tiger lily, American bistort, Indian paintbrush, and larkspur, are abundant, and the views are continuously outstanding. The final highlight comes in a huge meadow ▶5 on the slopes of a prominent rounded peak. From anywhere in this meadow, you'll have amazing views to the south and southwest of all the same canyons and peaks you have been enjoying all along, as well as a look down to the former Lake Mills, a reservoir that is now drained as part of the Elwha River restoration project. Given the crowds on Hurricane Hill, it is amazing that the view here, which is arguably just as good, is usually shared by just you and the marmots. After this meadow, the trail plunges

 Steep

 Wildflowers

 Viewpoint

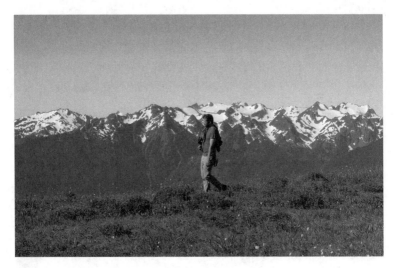

Hiker *atop Hurricane Hill*

thousands of feet down to a trailhead on the Elwha River. Unless you shuttled a car down there, however, the only sane thing to do is to return to the trailhead ▶6 the way you came.

🚶 MILESTONES

▶1	0.0	Trailhead (N47° 58.597' W123° 31.069')
▶2	0.3	Junction with Little River Trail (N47° 58.876' W123° 31.365')
▶3	1.4	Junction in meadow below summit (N47° 59.369' W123° 31.844')
▶4	1.6	Hurricane Hill (N47° 59.399' W123° 31.670')
▶5	3.4	Meadow viewpoint (N47° 57.297' W123° 50.092')
▶6	6.4	Return to trailhead (N47° 58.597' W123° 31.069')

Elk Mountain

Anchoring the western end of aptly named Grand Ridge, Elk Mountain offers some of the best views in Olympic National Park, which shouldn't be surprising because it features the highest maintained trail in the preserve. The "mountain" is really just a knob atop a long alpine ridge, and the trail doesn't even reach the official summit. But who really cares when the views from the trail itself are unsurpassed? And because the trailhead is already very high, you can reach these enchanting highlands after just a short (but steep) uphill. Once on the ridge, the walking is easy and about as close to hiking heaven as you can imagine.

Best Time

The trail is open from about mid-July to October. You will definitely want to wait for a clear day to enjoy the views. Avoid this trip in bad weather, as it is completely exposed to the elements and hypothermia is a real danger when conditions are wet, cold, and windy.

Finding the Trail

From US 101 in downtown Port Angeles, turn south on Race Street, following large signs pointing to Hurricane Ridge and Olympic National Park Visitor Center. This road eventually leaves town, becomes Mount Angeles Road, and passes the Olympic National Park Visitor Center and Wilderness Information Center on the right. At 1.2 miles from US 101 (or 0.1 mile past the visitor center), you bear

TRAIL USE
Day hiking,
child-friendly

LENGTH
5.0 miles, 2.5 hours

CUMULATIVE ELEVATION
730'

DIFFICULTY
- 1 2 **3** 4 5 +

TRAIL TYPE
Out-and-back

SURFACE TYPE
Dirt

CONTOUR MAP
Custom Correct
Hurricane Ridge

START & END
N47° 55.101'
W123° 22.930'

FEATURES
Mountain views,
abundant wildflowers

FACILITIES
Restrooms

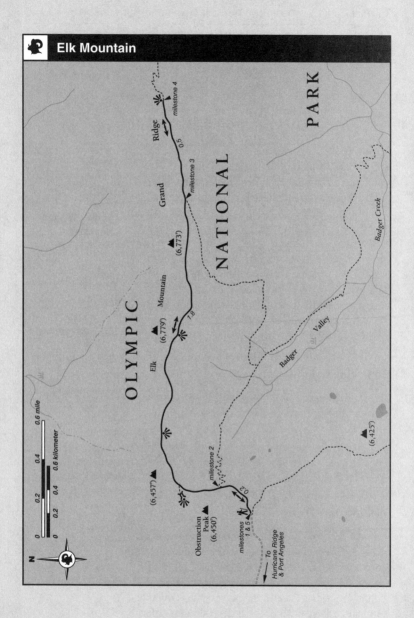

Elk Mountain

PARK

NATIONAL

OLYMPIC

Grand Ridge

milestone 4

0.5

milestone 3

(6,773')

1.8

Elk Mountain
(6,779')

(6,457')

milestone 2

Obstruction Peak
(6,450)

2.0

milestones
1 & 5

To
Hurricane Ridge
& Port Angeles

Badger Creek

Badger Valley

(6,425')

N

0   0.2   0.4   0.6 mile

0   0.2   0.4   0.6 kilometer

right at a prominent fork and then continue another 4.3 miles to the park's entrance station and pay booth. From here, climb the winding and increasingly scenic road for 12.5 miles to an easily missed junction immediately before the start of the large parking lot at the top of Hurricane Ridge.

You turn sharply left here on the narrow, gravel Obstruction Point Road. This road is fairly smooth at first, but it becomes much rougher (though still OK for passenger cars) after a couple of miles. You will reach the road-end trailhead after 7.8 miles.

Trail Description

Take the trail going east from the parking lot, ▶1 following signs to Grand Ridge and Deer Park. The route starts high and goes even higher, so while there is no shade, the views are terrific throughout.

The path begins by descending gently through rocky and rolling alpine terrain for a little more than 0.1 mile, and then it traverses the steep east side of Obstruction Peak. The path here is narrow and rocky, so watch your step to avoid a potentially nasty fall. Keeping your attention downward, however, is easier said than done because the views straight ahead of you to the long alpine ridge of Elk Mountain and down to your right of the green

 Viewpoint

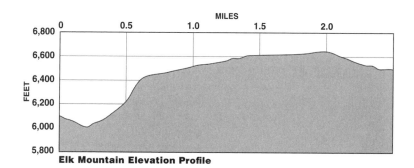

Elk Mountain Elevation Profile

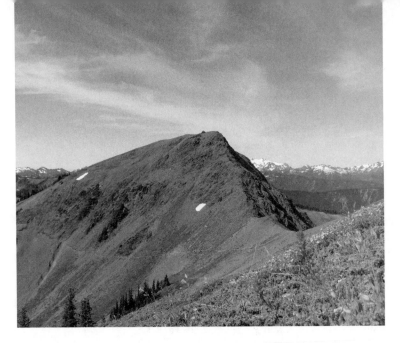

Obstruction Point *from Grand Ridge Trail on slopes of Elk Mountain*

expanse of Badger Valley tend to naturally draw your attention away from your feet.

At just more than 0.2 mile is a junction with the trail to Badger Valley ▶2 dropping to your right (see Trail 27). For this hike, go straight and continue the traverse of the steep slopes of Obstruction Peak. In some years, snowfields block this section until late July, so ask ahead about current conditions. The trail climbs a bit to a point just below a saddle on the northeast shoulder of Obstruction Peak. A short side trail climbs to the viewpoint at this pass. The trail then makes a steep uphill traverse of the south side of Elk Mountain. With all the trees below your elevation, the views are unobstructed and magnificent. The wildflowers are magnificent as well, with a wide variety of scattered but colorful species. Look for gentian, vetch, harebell, stonecrop, yarrow, larkspur, cinquefoil, Indian paintbrush, bistort, partridgefoot, owl's clover, and countless others.

As you gain elevation, the sights continue to improve, especially to the west where Mount

Steep

Viewpoint

Wildflowers

Olympus comes into view over the shoulder of Obstruction Peak. To the south, a whole array of tall peaks fills the skyline. At just short of 1 mile, the grade levels out as you cross the gentle and view-packed slopes just below the top of the ridge. It's a glorious and easy alpine walk, never surpassed and only rarely equaled in Olympic National Park. The trail rounds the slopes just below the official high point of Elk Mountain and then comes to a junction with the Elk Mountain Cutoff Trail ►**3**. This trail goes right on its way down to Badger Valley. From the area around this junction, you can see Grand Lake at the lower end of Grand Valley (see Trail 27).

You can turn around here, having already gathered more than enough memories to fill your vacation. The ridge walk continues, however, for another 5.5 miles, all the way to Deer Park. That's too far for most hikers, but at least save enough time and energy for the next 0.5 mile. This section remains high, with only a slight downhill grade, and offers many excellent views. Especially noteworthy are the vistas to the east of the distant Cascade Mountains and snow-covered volcanic peaks, such as Mount Baker and Glacier Peak. The logical turnaround point ►**4** is where the ridge gets narrow and the trail begins a long downhill to the saddle below Maiden Peak. Return to the parking lot ►**5** along the same alpine route you came in on, enjoying many of the same views but from the opposite direction.

 Viewpoint

![]	MILESTONES	
►1	0.0	Trailhead (N47° 55.101' W123° 22.930')
►2	0.2	Junction with Badger Valley Trail (N47° 55.249' W123° 22.790')
►3	2.0	Junction with Elk Mountain Cutoff Trail (N47° 55.407' W123° 20.849')
►4	2.5	Turnaround point on ridgetop (N47° 55.517' W123° 20.210')
►5	5.0	Return to trailhead (N47° 55.101' W123° 22.930')

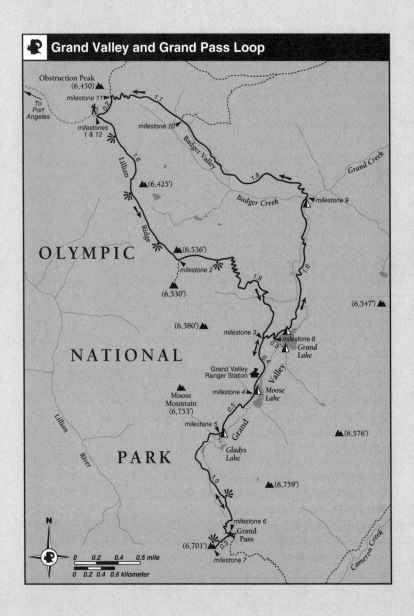

Grand Valley and Grand Pass Loop

Obstruction Peak
(6,450')

milestone 11

To Port Angeles

milestones 1 & 12

milestone 10

Badger Valley

Grand Creek

1.1

Lillian

1.6

(6,425')

Badger Creek

1.8

milestone 9

O L Y M P I C

Ridge

(6,536')

milestone 2

1.9

1.6

(6,547')

(6,530')

(6,580')

milestone 3

milestone 8

0.3

Grand
Lake

N A T I O N A L

Grand Valley
Ranger Station

0.4

Grand
Valley

Moose
Mountain
(6,753')

milestone 4

Moose
Lake

0.5

milestone 5

(6,576')

Lillian

Grand

Gladys
Lake

P A R K

River

1.5

(6,759')

N

milestone 6

Grand
Pass

(6,701')

0.3

Cameron Creek

milestone 7

0   0.2   0.4   0.5 mile

0   0.2 0.4 0.6 kilometer

Grand Valley and Grand Pass Loop

Grand is such an extreme superlative that only a handful of places in this country really qualify: Arizona's Grand Canyon and Wyoming's Grand Teton are at the top of the list. Perhaps not quite in the same league, but still *on* that list (which is really saying something), is Olympic National Park's Grand Valley. After a view-packed ramble along a high alpine ridge, the trail to this beauty spot plunges more than 1,600 feet down to the valley floor with its string of sparkling lakes, pretty stream, gorgeous meadows, and excellent campsites. Once in this mountain paradise, you can take a rugged but rewarding side trip to the stupendous viewpoint at Grand Pass before returning on a loop via the wildflower haven of Badger Valley.

To protect this much-visited area, the National Park Service has developed a limited number of designated campsites and employs a reservation system for overnight hiking between May 1 and September 30. Approximately half of the available camping spots are given out in reserved permits, with the remainder offered on a first-come, first-serve basis. To apply for a reservation, visit the park's website (**nps.gov/olym**), download a Wilderness Camping Permit Reservation Request form, fill out your information and planned itinerary, include your payment, and then send it by snail mail or fax (360-565-3108) to the Wilderness Information Center. Of course, strong day hikers can visit this area without worrying about a permit, but spending a night in this scenic masterpiece is well worth the extra effort.

TRAIL USE
Day hiking, backpacking

LENGTH
13.9 miles, 9 hours or 2–3 days (including Grand Pass side trip)

CUMULATIVE ELEVATION
4,100' (including Grand Pass side trip)

DIFFICULTY
- 1 2 3 4 **5** +

TRAIL TYPE
Loop

SURFACE TYPE
Dirt

CONTOUR MAP
Custom Correct *Hurricane Ridge* or *Elwha Valley*

START & END
N47° 55.101'
W123° 22.930'

FEATURES
Beautiful mountain lakes and meadows, views from both Lillian Ridge and Grand Pass, wildflowers in Badger Valley

FACILITIES
Restrooms

Best Time

The trail is often hikable by early July, but the access road typically does not melt out until mid-July. Call ahead or check the park's website for current conditions. Good weather allows you to better enjoy the scenery and have a much safer and more comfortable walk along Lillian Ridge at the start of the trip.

Finding the Trail

From US 101 in downtown Port Angeles, turn south on Race Street, following large signs pointing to Hurricane Ridge and Olympic National Park Visitor Center. This road eventually leaves town, becomes Mount Angeles Road, and passes the Olympic National Park Visitor Center and Wilderness Information Center on the right. At 1.2 miles from US 101 (or 0.1 mile past the visitor center), you bear right at a prominent fork and then continue another 4.3 miles to the park's entrance station and pay booth. From here, climb the winding and increasingly scenic road for 12.5 miles to an easily missed junction immediately before the start of the large parking lot at the top of Hurricane Ridge.

You turn sharply left here on the narrow, gravel Obstruction Point Road. This road is fairly smooth

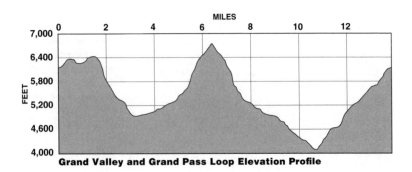

Grand Valley and Grand Pass Loop Elevation Profile

at first, but it becomes much rougher (though still OK for passenger cars) after a couple of miles. You'll reach the road-end trailhead after 7.8 miles.

Trail Description

Two trails begin from the Obstruction Point Trailhead. ►1 If you complete the loop, you will end up hiking both of them.

To start, take the trail going south–southeast toward Grand Valley. This path ascends a bit to the top of high, wide, and often windy Lillian Ridge, and then takes you on a top-of-the-world stroll across view-packed alpine terrain. The scenery is stupendous! Especially inspiring are the vistas to the west of the icy slopes of Mount Olympus and the Bailey Range. All that ice on those peaks, which are roughly the same elevation as you are, may make you wonder about the relative lack of snow and ice on Lillian Ridge. The two phenomena are actually connected. Because weather fronts typically come from the west in this region, the clouds hit those distant peaks first and drop most of their considerable moisture on those slopes. This leaves Lillian Ridge somewhat drier, benefiting from what is called the rain shadow effect.

Viewpoint

At about 0.6 mile, the trail descends to go around the west side of a rocky knoll. You then climb back up to the rolling ridgetop, passing high above several small ponds in the basins below the trail.

Near 1.6 miles, you reach the south side of a rounded high point in the ridge, where there is an unsigned but obvious junction with a use trail ►2 going south. If you just want a short day hike, this is a good turnaround point.

Those continuing with the loop should brace their knees because now comes a long and arduous downhill. The route is often steep, despite the 25 or so switchbacks put in to keep the grade reasonable.

Steep

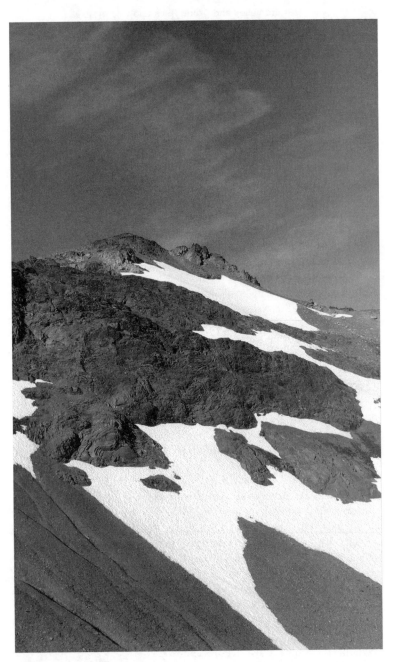

Ridge *west of trail up to Grand Pass*

The 1,600-foot descent begins on scree and tundra and then drops through open forest and meadows before entering denser forest. At the bottom is a junction ▶3 in a good-size meadow. Large and slightly green-tinged Grand Lake lies in the basin just below you.

The trail to the left is the recommended return route for the loop. But Grand Valley's best scenery is to the right. So turn that way and gradually climb in meadow and forest for 0.4 mile to the seasonal Grand Valley Ranger Station and, just beyond, Moose Lake. ▶4 Set beneath impressive peaks and surrounded by a mix of forest and flowery meadows, this is a beautiful place. Side trails lead to a number of excellent designated campsites, allowing you to enjoy this lake's charms at leisure.

Lake

Wildflowers

But Grand Valley isn't done with you just yet. So keep climbing, steeply at times, through increasingly open terrain. More campsites come along just before a short side trail goes left to shallow and meadow-rimmed Gladys Lake. ▶5 Above this small lake, the "grand" scenery continues, and even improves, as you pass meadows, ponds, and pretty little cascading waterfalls on your way back up into the alpine zone. The trail gets rockier and steeper as it winds its way up into a world of heather meadows and treeless slopes covered with talus and scree. Near the top, you pass an icy little snowmelt pond and just beyond come to Grand Pass. ▶6 Here, you are treated to excellent views, especially back down the way you came to Grand Valley and Moose Mountain. You can also look southwest to the rugged Cameron Pass area. For even broader views, take the unofficial trail that goes west from the pass and in 0.3 mile climbs steeply to the top of a 6,701-foot butte. ▶7 From here, you can see Mount Olympus, Mount Anderson, the remote Lillian River Valley, and even back to the Obstruction Point Trailhead. Turn around here, well satisfied with your efforts.

Lake

Waterfall

Steep

Viewpoint

Summit

To take the recommended loop trail on the way back, return to the junction above Grand Lake, go right (downhill), and descend five switchbacks to a junction beside large Grand Lake. ►8 The trail to the right goes to designated lakeside campsites.

Lake

You keep left, following the north shore of Grand Lake, and pass two more spur trails to inviting campsites. About 0.3 mile below the lake, you cross clear Grand Creek on a log bridge. Now entirely in forest, the trail goes mostly downhill, passing a hard-to-see waterfall along the way, and coming to a second log bridge over the creek just above a short waterfall and pool. You reach this loop's lowest elevation about 0.4 mile later at a log crossing of cascading Badger Creek. ►9 A good campsite is located about 100 yards before this crossing.

Waterfall

Now what you knew couldn't be put off forever finally begins: the long climb back to the trailhead. You have an intimidating 2,100 feet to gain, but on the plus side the grade is *usually* less severe than the route down from Lillian Ridge, which explains why this loop is recommended counterclockwise. You start in a shady forest as the trail switchbacks up a steep hillside. After about 0.5 mile, you leave the trees and enter a large, sloping meadow at the lower end of Badger Valley. There is no shade here, but you are compensated with abundant grasses and wildflowers waving in the breeze and nice views of the surrounding ridges and high points. Keep a sharp eye out for marmot holes as you walk through this meadow, as the animals seem to prefer the opening of the trail for their burrows. The continuous meadow ends in about 0.4 mile, after which you gradually climb through a mix of meadows and forests, making two crossings of a small creek along the way. Eventually, you reach the huge open meadows of upper Badger Valley, where there is a junction with the Elk Mountain Cutoff Trail. ►10

Steep

Wildflowers

Wildlife

Go straight at this junction and ascend increasingly scenic open slopes before finishing off the long climb with 16 steep switchbacks on a scree slope to a junction with Grand Ridge Trail. ▶11 Turn left and go gradually uphill across rocky alpine terrain for a little more than 0.2 mile back to the trailhead. ▶12

🚶 MILESTONES

▶1	0.0	Trailhead (N47° 55.101' W123° 22.930')
▶2	1.6	Junction with use trail (N47° 54.019' W123° 21.980')
▶3	3.5	Junction above Grand Lake (N47° 53.416' W123° 20.987')
▶4	3.9	Moose Lake (N47° 53.126' W123° 21.023')
▶5	4.4	Gladys Lake (N47° 52.701' W123° 21.537')
▶6	5.9	Grand Pass (N47° 51.939' W123° 21.373')
▶7	6.2	Butte 6701 (N47° 51.845' W123° 21.600')
▶8	9.2	Grand Lake (N47° 53.404' W123° 20.867')
▶9	10.8	Badger Creek (N47° 54.490' W123° 20.523')
▶10	12.6	Junction with Elk Mountain Cutoff (N47° 55.058' W123° 21.963')
▶11	13.7	Junction with Grand Ridge Trail (N47° 55.249' W123° 22.790')
▶12	13.9	Return to trailhead (N47° 55.101' W123° 22.930')

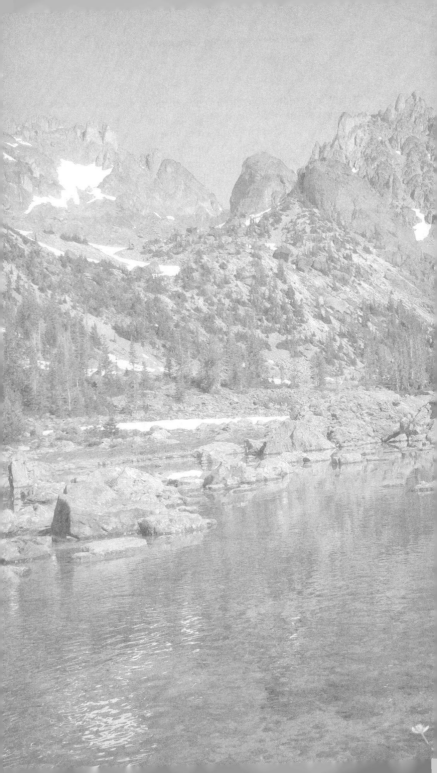

Northeast Region: The Rain Shadow Area

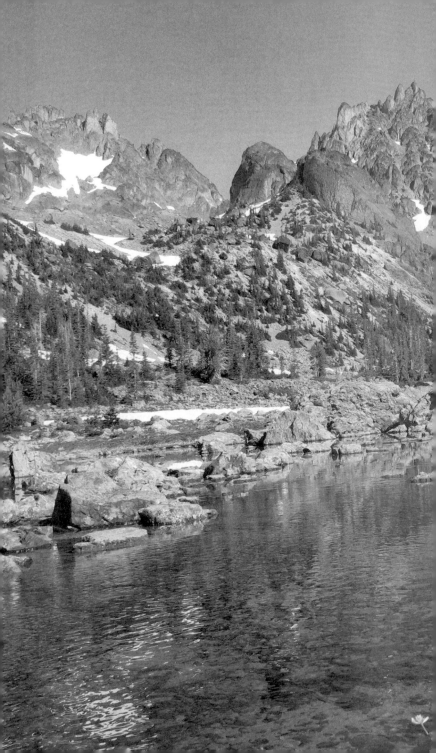

Northeast Region: The Rain Shadow Area

For a variety of reasons, the northeast region is my favorite hiking area on the Olympic Peninsula. First, and most obviously, the weather here is noticeably better than elsewhere on the peninsula. Sitting in the rain shadow of all those moisture-stealing peaks and ridges to the south and west, this area gets only a fraction of the rain and snow of other parts of the peninsula. The lowlands around the city of Sequim, for example, average a paltry 17 inches of precipitation per year, making this the driest and one of the sunniest places in all of western Washington. Hikes along the nearby Strait of Juan de Fuca are often wonderfully sunny, even while clouds and rain plague most other parts of the peninsula. And while the nearby mountains are a lot wetter than the lowlands, they are still much drier than the peaks to the west. As a result, the winter snows usually aren't as deep here and the trails melt out earlier in the hiking season.

The second great feature of this region is that you don't have to sacrifice scenery for improved weather. In fact, I would argue that the scenery here is perhaps the best on the entire peninsula. Excluding Mount Olympus, the peaks here are the highest in the range, and they are certainly more numerous and more jagged than most other parts of the Olympic Mountains. From every viewpoint, there are spiky peaks absolutely filling the skyline with their rugged beauty. In fact, in almost every way, the terrain here is more vertical and dramatic, with not just numerous steep-sided and jagged ridges and peaks, but also extremely deep canyons separating those ridges and wildly rushing streams cascading down the bottoms of the canyons.

The final point to make is that this region has practical advantages. If you are approaching from the Seattle metropolitan area, you will likely start by taking the ferry across Puget Sound to Edmonds. From there, it is only a short drive to the trails of the northeast region, making this the closest part of the Olympic Peninsula for people coming from that city.

Overleaf and opposite: *Mount Clark from Upper Royal Basin (Trail 31)*

Despite the area's many merits, most of the northeast region is not protected within the boundaries of Olympic National Park but instead is administered by the Olympic National Forest. With a different mandate, the US Forest Service manages the land differently than the national park. The forests are harvested here, so you may go through clear-cuts as you drive to the trailhead. Dogs are generally allowed on trails on national forest land, while they are prohibited in most of the park. Finally, hunting is allowed in the national forest, so the animals are usually more wary and you tend to see less wildlife than you do in the national park.

With the drier weather, the hiking season is somewhat longer in the northeast region than in other parts of the peninsula. The high-elevation, alpine trails here often melt out by mid-June rather than the norm of July or later in the mountains to the west. Also, in the winter, there is marginally less rain, snow, and ice at lower elevations here, so the trails are usually open and are often less muddy than winter trails in either the rain forest region or in areas to the south.

Note: More than 200 feet of the Dosewallips River Road was washed out by floods in 2002, which has left the last 5.5 miles of this important gravel thoroughfare closed to cars ever since. After much debate and public comment, the park has put forward a plan to rebuild and reopen this road to vehicle traffic. Unless and until this occurs, however, this section of road remains closed to cars but open to hikers. In the meantime, the extra road walk has placed several once-popular hikes, such as those to Lake Constance and Sunnybrook Meadows, out of the range of most day hikers, so they are not included in this book.

Governing Agencies

Dungeness Spit (Trail 28) falls under the management of Clallam County Parks and the Dungeness National Wildlife Refuge. Most of the hike to Royal Basin (Trail 31) and a portion of the hike to Baldy (Trail 30) are in Olympic National Park. All other trips in this region are administered by the Hood Canal Ranger District of Olympic National Forest.

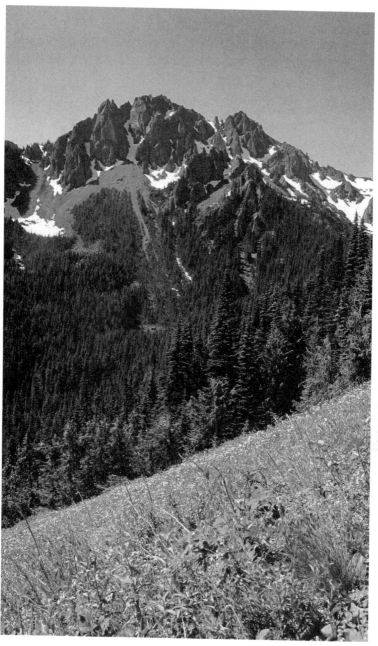

Along *Marmot Pass Trail below Camp Mystery (Trail 34)*

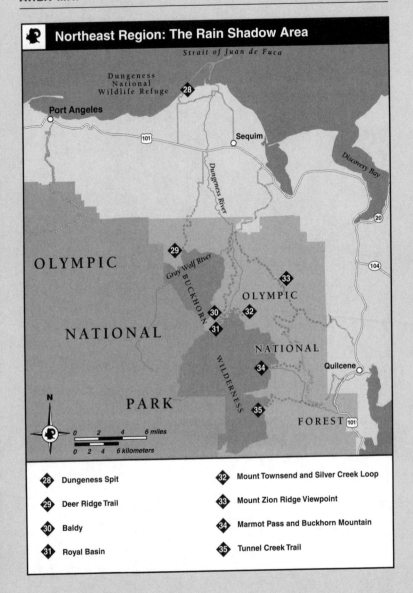

Northeast Region: The Rain Shadow Area

28 Dungeness Spit	**32** Mount Townsend and Silver Creek Loop
29 Deer Ridge Trail	**33** Mount Zion Ridge Viewpoint
30 Baldy	**34** Marmot Pass and Buckhorn Mountain
31 Royal Basin	**35** Tunnel Creek Trail

TRAIL FEATURES TABLE

Northeast Region: The Rain Shadow Area

TRAIL	DIFFICULTY	LENGTH	TYPE	USES & ACCESS	TERRAIN	FLORA & FAUNA	OTHER
28	3	10.8	Out-and-back	Day Hiking, Child-Friendly		Birds, Wildlife	Viewpoint, Historic Interest
29	4	10.2	Out-and-back	Day Hiking	Summit, Steep	Wildflowers, Wildlife	Viewpoint
30	5	8.2	Out-and-back	Day Hiking	Summit, Steep	Wildflowers	Viewpoint
31	4–5	14.0–15.8	Out-and-back	Day Hiking, Backpacking	Steep, Lake, Waterfall	Old-Growth Forest, Wildflowers	Viewpoint
32	5	7.6–10.9	Semi-loop	Day Hiking, Backpacking, Dogs Allowed	Summit, Steep, Lake	Wildflowers	Viewpoint, Geologic Interest
33	3	4.6	Out-and-back	Day Hiking, Mountain Biking, Horses, Dogs Allowed, Child-Friendly	Summit, Steep	Wildflowers	Viewpoint
34	5	10.6–12.4	Out-and-back	Day Hiking, Backpacking, Horses, Dogs Allowed	Summit, Steep, Waterfall	Old-Growth Forest, Wildflowers, Wildlife	Viewpoint
35	4	9.2	Out-and-back	Day Hiking, Backpacking, Dogs Allowed	Steep, Lake	Old-Growth Forest, Wildflowers	Viewpoint, Historic Interest

USES & ACCESS
- Day Hiking
- Backpacking
- Mountain Biking
- Horses
- Dogs Allowed
- Child-Friendly

TYPE
- Loop
- Semi-loop
- Out-and-back

DIFFICULTY
- 1 2 3 4 5 +
less   more

TERRAIN
- Summit
- Steep
- Lake
- Waterfall
- Tidepool

FLORA & FAUNA
- Old-Growth Forest
- Wildflowers
- Birds
- Wildlife

OTHER
- Viewpoint
- Geologic Interest
- Historic Interest

Northeast Region: The Rain Shadow Area

Dungeness Spit is the longest coastal spit in the continental United States, and the lighthouse at the end of this long and narrow peninsula of sand makes for a terrific hiking destination. The views are wonderful, the wildlife (especially birds) is plentiful, and the lighthouse is a fascinating and very photogenic location. Because the walking is mostly level and on hard-packed sand, this hike is not terribly difficult, even though it is rather long. Try to visit on a calm day in the off-season to avoid two common problems: wind and crowds.

One of the best early-summer hikes in the range, this trail climbs a rhododendron-covered ridge to a series of outstanding overlooks featuring fine views of a wealth of snowy mountains and deep canyons. In late June, before the road to Deer Park opens and the crowds arrive, this trail is the perfect combination of solitude, wildflowers, scenery, and wildlife (mostly deer, as the name of the ridge suggests).

Strictly for experienced and well-conditioned hikers, this exhausting and extremely steep trail leads to arguably the best viewpoint on the entire Olympic Peninsula. The views of Royal Basin, the Dungeness River canyon, the extremely rugged Gray Wolf Divide, and distant Mount Olympus, among other landmarks, are truly jaw dropping. Thus, all those sore muscles and jammed toes you'll be nursing for the next several days will be compensated by great pictures and fine memories. But only you can decide if the experience is worth the effort.

Royal Basin 260

TRAIL 31

This is a long and deservedly popular trail to an idyllic mountain basin set directly beneath some of the tallest and most spectacular peaks in the Olympic Mountains. The popularity has forced the National Park Service to require that all overnight visitors obtain advanced reservations for the limited number of available backcountry permits. Strong day hikers, however, can do the trip without any permit hassles, and those lucky backpackers with an overnight permit can extend their outing to an upper alpine wonderland with some of the most dramatic mountain scenery in the entire park.

Day hiking,
backpacking
14.0–15.8 miles
Out-and-back
Difficulty: 1 2 3 **4 5**

Mount Townsend and Silver Creek Loop 266

TRAIL 32

Mount Townsend is, justly, one of the most well-liked viewpoint hikes in the Olympic Mountains. The scenery from this alpine grandstand is truly breathtaking. The route to the top described here, however, is so off the beaten track and rarely hiked that you may be alone on the trail (though not on the summit). It's a steep and tiring climb, however, so be prepared. For backpackers and *really* strong day hikers, a loop is possible that includes a gorgeous little mountain lake and a return route along an unofficial and rugged way trail beside the rollicking waters of a pretty mountain stream.

Day hiking, backpacking, mountain biking, horses, dogs allowed
7.6–10.9 miles
Out-and-back/Loop
Difficulty: 1 2 3 4 **5**

Mount Zion Ridge Viewpoint 274

TRAIL 33

Mount Zion may be the best place in Washington to enjoy the bright pink blossoms of the state flower, the Pacific rhododendron. In mid- to late June, you'll be treated to acres of color. And for extra bonus points, the view from a rocky outcrop along the ridge a little beyond the summit would make this hike worthwhile even without the flowers.

Day hiking, dogs allowed, child-friendly
4.6 miles
Out-and-back
Difficulty: 1 2 **3** 4 5

TRAIL 34

Marmot Pass and Buckhorn Mountain 280

A favorite of generations of hikers, the diverse and very scenic trail up to Marmot Pass along the Big Quilcene River features everything the Olympic Mountains have to offer in one impressive package. Here, you'll be treated to lots of wildflowers, dense forests, a lively mountain stream, good campsites, the potential for wildlife sightings, and, from the pass, stupendous views of some of the tallest and most rugged peaks in the range. Marmot Pass is far enough for most, but those with more endurance can extend their outing to an even higher observation point on the slopes of nearby Buckhorn Mountain.

TRAIL 35

Tunnel Creek Trail 286

Early in the season, this trip can be done as a fairly easy and very enjoyable forest ramble along an enchanting mountain stream. Once summer comes along, however, you can continue your hike by climbing to a shallow little lake and a terrific ridgetop overlook with the best view anywhere of towering Mount Constance, one of the highest peaks in the Olympic Mountains.

Dungeness Spit

Dungeness Spit, the longest coastal spit in the continental United States, is a narrow peninsula of sand that extends almost 6 miles into the Strait of Juan de Fuca. Because it juts so far out into a busy shipping lane, the place is a natural location for a lighthouse, and the one sitting near the end of the spit makes an excellent hiking destination at any time of year. The peninsula is protected as a national wildlife refuge, so it's not surprising that there is also a lot of wildlife here to spot. Deer are extremely common along the short forest walk to the start of the spit, and birds are everywhere. You will see a wide variety of seabirds, and bald eagles are particularly abundant. Most visitors see several eagles during the course of their hike. The star attraction, however, is the lovingly restored and exceptionally photogenic lighthouse. Tours are provided by a group of dedicated volunteer lighthouse enthusiasts, and the views from the top of the tower are terrific.

Best Time

The trail and beach route are open all year, and the hike is fun in any season. It can be crowded, however, so for seclusion and better wildlife viewing, choose a weekday in the off-season. It can be very windy on this exposed spit, so visit on a calm day. Clear skies allow you to enjoy nice views of the Olympic Mountains, but the hike is pleasurable in almost any weather. Low tide is not required, but it does make the hiking somewhat easier as you will be able to do most of your walking on hard-packed sand.

TRAIL USE
Day hiking,
child-friendly

LENGTH
10.8 miles, 5 hours

CUMULATIVE ELEVATION
125'

DIFFICULTY
- 1 2 **3** 4 5 +

TRAIL TYPE
Out-and-back

SURFACE TYPE
Pavement, sand

CONTOUR MAP
None needed (you couldn't get lost if you wanted to).

START & END
N48° 08.486'
W123° 11.446'

FEATURES
Long coastal sand spit, excellent views, lighthouse, abundant wildlife

FACILITIES
Restrooms, picnic tables, water

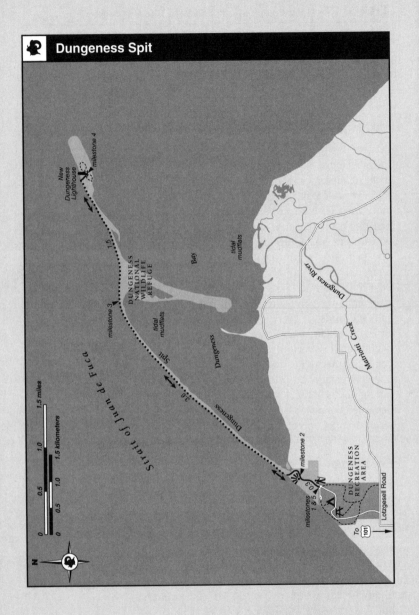

Dungeness Spit

New Dungeness Lighthouse

milestone 4

milestone 3

DUNGENESS NATIONAL WILDLIFE REFUGE

1.5

Bay

tidal mudflats

tidal mudflats

Strait of Juan de Fuca

Dungeness Spit

tidal mudflats

Dungeness

Dungeness River

0.5

milestone 2

Mariatti Creek

milestones 1 & 5

0.3

DUNGENESS RECREATION AREA

Lotzgesell Road

To 101

N

0   0.5   1.0   1.5 miles

0   0.5   1.0   1.5 kilometers

Finding the Trail

Leave US 101 at milepost 260 about 11 miles east of Port Angeles. Turn north on paved Kitchen-Dick Road, following signs to Dungeness Recreation Area, and drive 1.5 miles to a four-way stop. Go straight and drive another 1.8 miles to the point where the road makes a 90-degree turn to the right (east) and becomes Lotzgesell Road. Just 0.2 mile after this turn, you come to the well-signed entrance road for the Dungeness Wildlife and Recreation Area. You turn left and almost immediately pass through a gate that automatically closes at 10 p.m. and opens again at 7 a.m. Drive 0.8 mile to a fee booth for people staying at the campground, and then proceed past various side roads that lead to picnic areas and campground loops, always following signs to the trailhead and day-use area. About 0.3 mile from the fee booth is the large trailhead parking lot.

Trail Description

The trail departs from the northeast end of the parking lot ▶1 near a cluster of large signboards. You initially wander through a relatively dry (by Olympic standards), mostly coniferous forest with the usual Douglas-firs, western hemlocks, and western red cedars. The forest also includes some Pacific madrones, which is solid evidence of the dryness of this moss-free rain shadow forest. Salal dominates the crowded forest floor. The path is wide and paved as it very gradually descends through the shady forest. For much of the year, the songs of birds are added to the sound of distant waves for a pleasant mix of audio stimulation. At 0.3 mile is a wooden viewing platform ▶2 overlooking the harbor and the long, narrow curve of Dungeness Spit. You now make a well-graded descent to the end of the paved trail, where it meets the beach on the north side of the spit. Early in the morning, it is common to see deer

Viewpoint

Wildlife

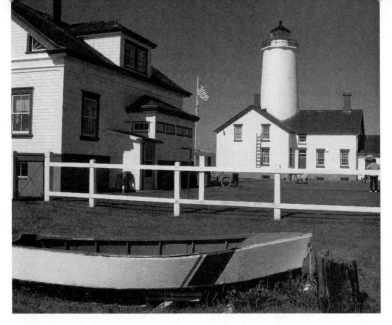

Old boat *and New Dungeness Lighthouse*

on the beach here, often lapping at the ocean water for the salt.

Turn right (northeast) and begin walking the long strip of sand. Be sure to look behind you from time to time for nice views of a cluster of craggy peaks in the Olympic Mountains near Hurricane Ridge. Piles of drift logs line the inland side of the beach route. To protect the nesting areas of birds, refuge regulations prohibit visitor access to the drift logs and the bay side of the spit, so please stay on the narrow strip of hikable sand on the northwest side of the peninsula.

The hike is fairly long but perfectly straightforward as you simply follow the sand, listening to the gently lapping waves and looking for assorted seabirds along the way. The walking, especially at low tide, is easy, generally on stable, fairly hard-packed sand. The spit gradually curves to the east, providing continuous views of the wide Strait of Juan de Fuca; the distant hills and mountains of Vancouver Island; and, on really clear days, the towering white pyramid

Viewpoint

of Mount Baker in the Cascade Mountains. Also of interest are the constant stream of oceangoing cargo and navy ships carrying goods and sailors to and from the ports of Seattle and Vancouver to and from all parts of the world. Another thing to occupy your attention are bald eagles, several of which are often seen flying overhead or perched on drift logs.

Birds

At around 3.9 miles, at a prominent curve in the spit, ▶3 your destination comes into view, the squat lighthouse near the tip of Dungeness Spit. The lighthouse seems to grow in stature as you get closer, with its white tower rising above the nearby outbuildings to a height of 67 feet.

Once you reach the photogenic lighthouse ▶4 at 5.4 miles, take some time to explore the grounds and walk the nearby interpretive trails that display the history of this place. Volunteers offer interesting tours of the lighthouse, starting at 9 a.m. as visitors show up. Donations are gladly accepted, as the maintenance of this historic structure is in the hands of a nonprofit organization. The lighthouse even provides a drinking fountain, which is fed, of all things, by a freshwater artesian well at the end of this low spit surrounded by saltwater.

Historic Interest

To protect the wildlife, access to the actual end of the spit beyond the lighthouse is prohibited, so enjoy the historic structure and return along the sand to the trailhead ▶5 the way you came.

🚶	**MILESTONES**		
▶1	0.0	Take trail from parking lot (N48° 08.486' W123° 11.446')
▶2	0.3	Viewing platform (N48° 08.737' W123° 11.165')
▶3	3.9	Curve in spit toward lighthouse (N48° 10.526' W123° 08.758')
▶4	5.4	New Dungeness Lighthouse (N48° 10.908' W123° 06.602')
▶5	10.8	Return to trailhead (N48° 08.486' W123° 11.446')

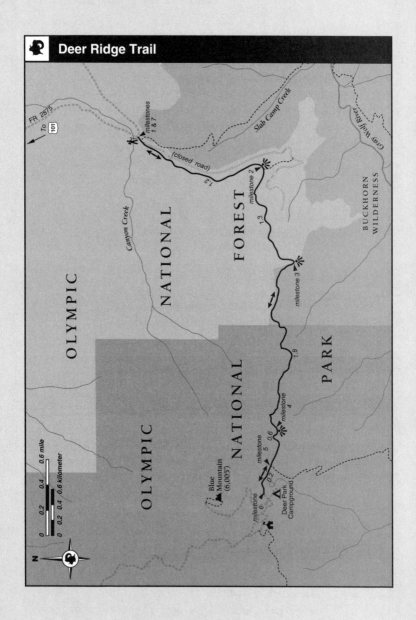

Deer Ridge Trail

milestones
1 & 7

Slab Camp Creek

FR 2875

To 101

(closed road)

1.2

milestone 2

1.3

Gray Wolf River

BUCKHORN
WILDERNESS

Canyon Creek

NATIONAL

FOREST

milestone 3

1.8

PARK

OLYMPIC

NATIONAL

milestone
4

0.6

milestone
5

0.2

OLYMPIC

Blue
Mountain
(6,005')

milestone
6

Deer Park
Campground

N

0   0.2   0.4   0.6 mile

0   0.2   0.4   0.6 kilometer

Deer Ridge Trail

Deer Park is a busy, high-elevation destination in the northeast corner of Olympic National Park. July–October the park can be reached by a steep and winding gravel road. Locals know, however, that you can also reach this mountain paradise before the road opens via a quiet trail that climbs to the area from US Forest Service land to the east. In fact, on a sunny day in late June, it is hard to imagine a more scenic hiking destination on the entire peninsula. The trip involves a stiff climb, so it's not for everyone, but for wildflowers, wildlife, and outstanding mountain views, it's hard to beat.

Best Time

The trail is usually hikable June–October. Mid- to late June is ideal for blooming rhododendrons at lower elevations and rock-garden wildflowers up high. The road to Deer Park usually opens in early July, so mid- to late June will also ensure having the high country to yourself. Photo and wildlife-viewing opportunities are better in the morning.

Finding the Trail

Drive US 101 to a junction near milepost 262, about 1 mile west of Sequim. Turn south on Taylor Cutoff Road, go 5.4 miles on this paved road, and then turn left onto gravel Slab Camp Road. After 0.9 mile, you fork right onto Forest Road 2875 and proceed 3.7 miles to a large gravel pullout and trailhead on the right.

TRAIL USE
Day hiking

LENGTH
10.2 miles, 5 hours

CUMULATIVE ELEVATION
2,840'

DIFFICULTY
- 1 2 3 **4** 5 +

TRAIL TYPE
Out-and-back

SURFACE TYPE
Dirt

CONTOUR MAP
Custom Correct *Gray Wolf–Dosewallips*

START & END
N47° 57.897'
W123° 11.593'

FEATURES
Mountain scenery, rhododendrons, alpine wildflowers, abundant wildlife

FACILITIES
None

Trail Description

The trail initially goes south from the parking lot ►1 on an old gravel road that is now closed to vehicles. After only 15 yards, the trail splits. Go straight on Deer Ridge Trail and very gradually ascend a forested hillside above the old road. There are frequent nice views to the south of snowy Tyler Peak and Baldy. In the latter half of June, blooming rhododendrons put on a terrific display of color along this section of the trail. At about 0.8 mile, the pace of your ascent goes from gentle to moderately steep; at 1.2 miles, you round a prominent ridge and come to a nice open viewpoint. ►2 The broad summit of Baldy (Trail 30) fills the sky to the south and towers above the green depths of the Gray Wolf River Canyon.

About 40 yards after this point, you go straight where an unsigned and now abandoned trail goes left and downhill. The main trail continues climbing, generally remaining in the welcome shade of dense forest. At about 1.7 miles is another rocky outcrop on your left with nice views, though this time the scenery is partially blocked by trees. The trail then goes up a much steeper section before reaching a third viewpoint on another spur ridge. ►3 To the south–southwest rise the rugged high peaks of the Gray Wolf Divide, while to the west

Wildflowers

Steep

Steep

Viewpoint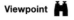

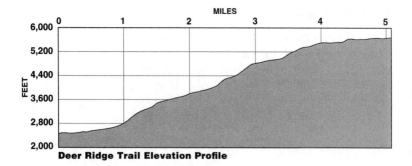

Deer Ridge Trail Elevation Profile

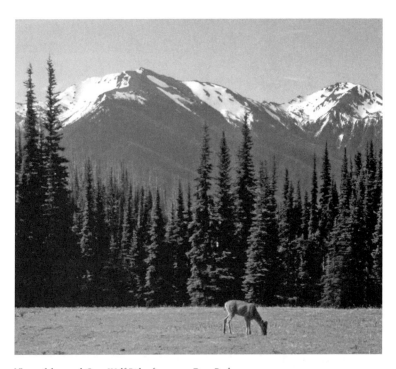

View *of deer and Gray Wolf Ridge from near Deer Park*

and west–southwest are an arc of snowy summits around Cameron Pass and the headwaters of the Gray Wolf River. It's a marvelous scene, and for a comfortable way to take it all in, walk about 50 yards up the trail to a couple of benches, where you can sit and admire the view. These benches were installed by a local hiking club in memory of former club members who helped to maintain this wonderful trail.

The trail turns right at the viewpoint, steeply climbing the spine of the spur ridge, where short trees, twisted by frequent high winds, provide excellent frames for photographs of the distant mountains. After only 0.1 mile, the trail angles to

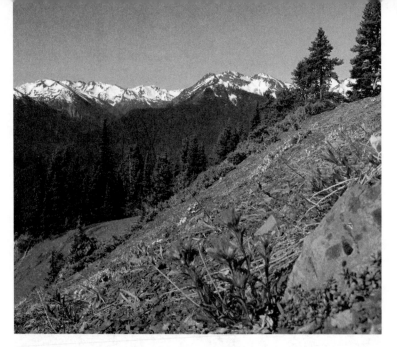

Paintbrush *and view west from upper reaches of Deer Ridge Trail*

Viewpoint

the left off the ridge and crosses a partially forested slope with frequent outstanding views over the Gray Wolf Valley and its surrounding peaks. At a couple of points, you will even catch glimpses to the east of Puget Sound and Glacier Peak in the Cascade Range.

At about 3.8 miles, you reach the top of Deer Ridge with its spire-shaped subalpine firs and scrubby lodgepole pines. The ridge also features numerous wildflower-covered meadows, awesome

Wildlife

views, and, yes, high concentrations of deer. It is common to see a dozen or more feeding in the meadows here, especially early in the morning. The trail enters Olympic National Park in this vicinity, though there is no sign at the boundary.

The trail soon cuts back over to the view-packed south side of the ridge and keeps climbing, though

Viewpoint

now at a very gentle grade. At about 4.3 miles, you come to a wonderful viewpoint ►4 with wide vistas over more peaks, ridges, and canyons than I could possibly list. In late June there are also a wealth of tiny rock-garden wildflowers here, including Indian paintbrush, spreading phlox, smooth douglasia, grass widow, and Lomatium.

 Wildflowers

The hiking is now easy and scenic as you contour across open slopes for 0.6 mile to a junction. ▶5 The trail to the left drops to Three Forks and the Gray Wolf River. Keep straight and walk on a virtually level trail for a little more than 0.2 mile on the open southern slopes of Blue Mountain to a gravel turnaround and trailhead parking area off Deer Park Road. ▶6 If you've had your fill of mountain scenery, turn around here and return to the trailhead. ▶7 If you are still bursting with energy, however, you can continue the hike by walking up the gravel road to the nature trails around the summit of Blue Mountain with its 360-degree views.

 Summit

Tip: If you want a very easy hike, wait until Deer Park Road opens, drive to the upper trailhead, and simply walk the easy and mostly level 0.8 mile to the high viewpoint noted above.

🚶 MILESTONES

▶1	0.0	Take trail from parking lot (N47° 57.897' W123° 11.593')
▶2	1.2	First viewpoint (N47° 56.966' W123° 11.913')
▶3	2.5	Third viewpoint (N47° 56.746' W123° 12.968')
▶4	4.3	Ridge viewpoint (N47° 56.804' W123° 14.740')
▶5	4.9	Three Forks junction (N47° 56.893' W123° 15.193')
▶6	5.1	Deer Park Road (N47° 56.941' W123° 15.497')
▶7	10.2	Return to trailhead (N47° 57.897' W123° 11.593')

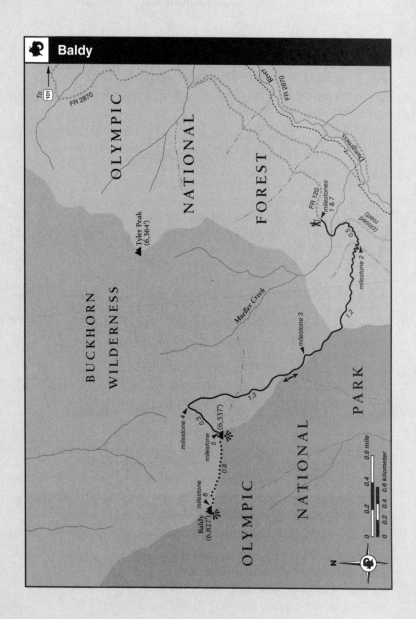

Baldy

OLYMPIC NATIONAL FOREST

To 101
FR 2870

Tyler Peak
(6,364')

BUCKHORN WILDERNESS

Mueller Creek

FR 2870
River

Dungeness

FR 120
milestones
1 & 7

(closed road)

0.5

milestone 2

1.2

milestone 3

1.3

milestone 4

0.3

milestone 5
(6,537')

0.8

milestone 6

Baldy
(6,827')

OLYMPIC NATIONAL PARK

N

0   0.2   0.4   0.6 mile

0   0.2   0.4   0.6 kilometer

Baldy

Before I give all the usual glowing reports about how beautiful this hike is, I feel obligated to say that most readers should probably forget all that and not take this trip. There's no two ways about it—this is a *punishing* hike on a ridiculously steep trail that will really test your lungs and thighs on the way up. And you won't get a break on the way back down either because your knees and toes will surely complain about all the pounding and jamming. Also, on the descent, you will need to be very careful with your footing to avoid a fall at places with loose pebbles. Thus, only the strongest and most sure-footed hikers should take this trip.

So why, you reasonably ask, did I include it in this book? Because this killer trail provides arguably the best killer views on the entire Olympic Peninsula, and if you've already hiked some of the other trails in this book, you'll realize what incredibly high praise that is. In other words, even though you will almost certainly be tired and sore after this hike, you won't be disappointed.

Best Time

The trail is usually open from very late June to October. Mid-July is ideal for alpine wildflowers. Definitely save this for a clear day, but not one that is too hot, because the climb is tough enough without the heat.

TRAIL USE
Day hiking

LENGTH
8.2 miles, 5-6 hours

CUMULATIVE ELEVATION
3,900'

DIFFICULTY
- 1 2 3 4 **5** +

TRAIL TYPE
Out-and-back

SURFACE TYPE
Dirt

CONTOUR MAP
Green Trails *Tyler Peak* #136 or Custom Correct *Buckhorn Wilderness*

START & END
N47° 52.944'
W123° 08.603'

FEATURES
Views over the most rugged and dramatic peaks, canyons, and ridges in the Olympic Mountains; wildflowers; tough climb

FACILITIES
None

255

Finding the Trail

Leave US 101 about 1.5 miles east of Sequim near milepost 267.2 at a junction just southeast of the turnoff for John Wayne Marina. Turn south on Palo Alto Road and follow this good, paved, county road for 8.3 miles to a road fork, where signs point right to Dungeness Forks Campground. Bear right (downhill) on Forest Road 2880 and drive 1.7 miles on this narrow gravel road to a prominent junction with FR 2870. Go left here, following signs to Dungeness Trail, and proceed 2.6 miles to another major junction. Keep right, still on FR 2870, and drive 4.9 miles to a junction with a minor side road that angles off to the right. This is FR 120, though there will probably not be a sign to that effect. There usually is, however, a small sign here pointing to Maynard Burn Trail. Go right and slowly drive 1.8 miles to the road-end turnaround and trailhead. These last 1.8 miles are narrow and a bit rough but drivable with a passenger car. The old road beyond this point is washed out and blocked off. There is parking for about four cars at this small and primitive trailhead.

Trail Description

From the small trailhead parking area, ▶1 you go southwest, initially staying mostly level as you follow

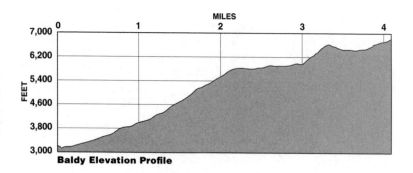

Baldy Elevation Profile

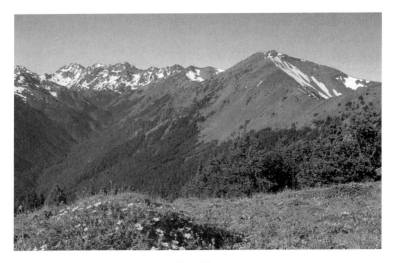

Looking south *toward Royal Basin area from false summit*

the continuation of the long-abandoned and now mostly overgrown road. This route soon takes you to Mueller Creek, where you make an easy rock-hop crossing. About 150 yards after this crossing, look for a well-traveled trail angling to the right. This route is usually marked with an orange flag. Turn onto this trail and soon begin the promised climb, which gains an absurd 2,100 feet in the next 1.5 miles.

The climb begins easily enough on a steep, but not yet extremely steep, route through an open forest of western hemlocks and Douglas-firs. After 0.3 mile, you come to another junction with the old gravel road. ▶2 After a brief jog to the right, the path, now called Maynard Burn Trail, continues uphill on the other side of the road. And when I say uphill, I *really* mean uphill. Switchbacks, you ask? Nope, say the trail builders. We don't need no stinking switchbacks. We learned in geometry class that the shortest distance between two points is a straight line, and that's good enough for us. Fortunately, trees provide

Steep

very welcome shade, but your leg and butt muscles will still get a real workout. The path generally remains near the top of a rounded ridge and heads northwest, though the dominant direction of travel is vertical, not horizontal.

The forest gradually thins out as you ascend with increasing numbers of lodgepole pines, Pacific silver firs, and even a few western white pines, the last an unusual species in the Olympic Mountains. At about 1.7 miles, just before an anomalous little flat spot, ▶3 the trail makes a jog to the left and resumes climbing, albeit at a somewhat more reasonable grade. Very soon thereafter, you pass an easy-to-miss marker at the border of Olympic National Park. Things become easier about 0.4 mile later when the trail angles to the right, leaving the ridge, and after a bit more uphill actually remains nearly level for about 0.2 mile as it traverses a steep open slope with excellent views and lots of wildflowers. The best views are to the south–southeast of the area around Buckhorn Mountain and Warrior Peak. July-blooming wildflowers in this sloping meadow include bistort, buttercup, aster, phlox, lupine, larkspur, arnica, and woolly yellow daisy. Steep climbing resumes at the north side of this open slope as the sometimes faint path rapidly ascends the edge of the meadow to the top of a ridge ▶4 between Baldy and Tyler Peak. Views from here are excellent, especially looking north to Vancouver Island.

You won't want to stop hiking just yet, however, because the best views are still to come. So turn left and follow a very steep intermittent boot path that climbs a grassy and rocky slope for about 0.3 mile to the top of a false summit of Baldy. ▶5 And BOOM, conclusive evidence that the Ringling Brothers have it wrong: They are *not* the greatest show on Earth. The all-natural show you are treated to here is jaw-droppingly amazing, as it better be, after your body paid such a high-ticket price. The most dramatic scene is looking south to tall Mount Deception,

Viewpoint

Wildflowers

Steep

Summit

Viewpoint

jagged Gray Wolf Ridge, aptly named The Needles, and the deep bowl of Royal Basin. Other outstanding scenes are to the west of nearby Baldy and the top of distant and glacier-clad Mount Olympus; southwest to Mount Constance and its surrounding peaks; north to the Port Angeles lowlands, the Strait of Juan de Fuca, and Vancouver Island; northeast to the volcanic cone of Mount Baker; and east to the Puget Sound area and the Cascade Range. Views simply don't get much better than this.

You could spend hours here resting (you'll need the rest) and soaking in the view, but if you want to do more exploring, the actual summit of Baldy makes an excellent and obvious goal. To reach it, follow the ridge to the west as it drops about 150 feet to a saddle and then ascends rocky terrain and grassy tundra to Baldy's rounded top. ▶6 The views aren't any better here than at the false summit (they couldn't be), but you do have a better perspective to the west of the Hurricane Ridge area, the deep canyons of the three main branches of the Gray Wolf River, and Mount Olympus. After taking in all the scenery, figuratively put on a pair of knee braces (or literally, if you have them) and tackle the return trip to the trailhead. ▶7

 Summit

 Viewpoint

 	MILESTONES	
▶1	0.0	Start at road-end trailhead (N47° 52.944' W123° 08.603')
▶2	0.5	Cross old gravel road (N47° 52.741' W123° 08.797')
▶3	1.7	Small flat spot (N47° 53.070' W123° 09.877')
▶4	3.0	Ridge crest (N47° 53.758' W123° 10.460')
▶5	3.3	False summit (N47° 53.638' W123° 10.612')
▶6	4.1	Baldy summit (N47° 53.701' W123° 11.356')
▶7	8.2	Return to trailhead (N47° 52.944' W123° 08.603')

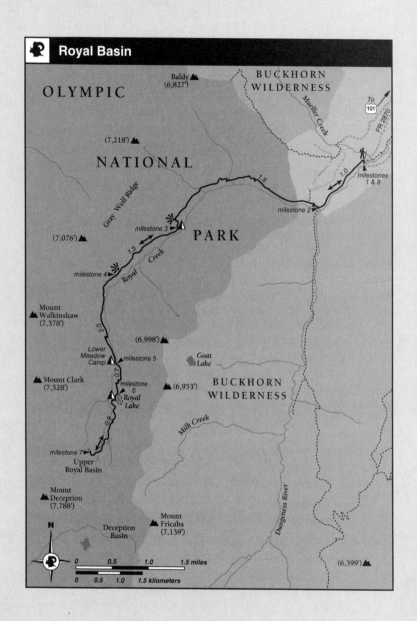

OLYMPIC

Baldy
(6,827')

BUCKHORN
WILDERNESS

Mueller Creek

To
101

FR 2870

(7,218')

NATIONAL

1.8

1.0

milestones
1 & 8

Gray Wolf Ridge

milestone 3

PARK

milestone 2

(7,076')

1.5

Royal Creek

milestone 4

Mount
Walkinshaw
(7,378')

0.2

(6,998')

Goat
Lake

Lower
Meadow
Camp

milestone 5

BUCKHORN
WILDERNESS

Mount Clark
(7,528')

0.2

milestone
6
Royal
Lake

(6,953')

Milk Creek

0.9

milestone 7

Upper
Royal Basin

Mount
Deception
(7,788')

Dungeness River

N

Deception
Basin

Mount
Fricaba
(7,139')

0   0.5   1.0   1.5 miles

0   0.5   1.0   1.5 kilometers

(6,599')

Royal Basin

A more than suitable playground for even the most finicky monarch, Royal Basin is a multileveled alpine bowl that sits directly beneath some of the tallest, most rugged, and most beautiful peaks in the Olympic Mountains. The outstanding scenery here has drawn legions of admirers for decades, so don't expect to be alone. To protect this area from overuse, the National Park Service requires a limited-use permit for all overnight travel into the basin between May 1 and September 30. These permits are available *by reservation only* (no first-come, first-serve permits are set aside) and must be obtained from the Wilderness Information Center in Port Angeles. To apply for a reservation, visit the park's website (**nps.gov/olym**), download a Wilderness Camping Permit Reservation Request form, fill out your information and planned itinerary, include your payment, and then send it by snail mail or fax (360-565-3108) to the Wilderness Information Center. Well-conditioned day hikers, however, can reach this beautiful goal without any permit hassles and can travel on the spur of the moment.

Best Time

The trail as far as Royal Lake is usually open July–October. Upper Royal Basin is not typically free of snow until at least mid-July. Late July is ideal because there will still be some wildflowers along the lower trail, snow will still be streaking the high peaks for better scenery, and the first blossoms will be coming in as the snow melts at high elevations. If you are doing this as a day hike, then get an early

TRAIL USE
Day hiking, backpacking

LENGTH
14.0 miles, 7 hours or overnight (to Royal Lake); 15.8 miles, 2 days (to Upper Royal Basin)

CUMULATIVE ELEVATION
2,500' (to Royal Lake); 3,150' (to Upper Royal Basin)

DIFFICULTY
- 1 2 3 **4 5** +

TRAIL TYPE
Out-and-back

SURFACE TYPE
Dirt

CONTOUR MAP
Green Trails *Tyler Peak* #136 or Custom Correct *Buckhorn Wilderness*

START & END
N47° 52.651'
W123° 08.221'

FEATURES
Mountain scenery and views, pretty mountain lake, abundant wildflowers, lower-elevation forests and streams

FACILITIES
Restrooms

261

start; it is a long trip, and you will need plenty of time to savor the scenery.

Finding the Trail

Leave US 101 about 1.5 miles east of Sequim near milepost 267.2 at a junction just southeast of the turnoff for John Wayne Marina. Turn south on Palo Alto Road and follow this good, paved, county road for 8.3 miles to a road fork, where signs point right to Dungeness Forks Campground. Bear right (downhill) on Forest Road 2880 and drive 1.7 miles on this narrow gravel road to a prominent junction with FR 2870. Go left here, following signs to Dungeness Trail, and proceed 2.6 miles to another major junction. Keep right, still on FR 2870, and drive 6.6 miles to the large Dungeness Trailhead parking area on the right just after a bridge over the Dungeness River.

Trail Description

Old-Growth Forest

Leave the parking lot ▸1 and walk back across the road bridge to the signed trailhead on the west side of the river. After one quick switchback, the trail turns south (upstream), traveling through a beautiful and relatively open old-growth forest close to the clear Dungeness River. The path has some ups and downs

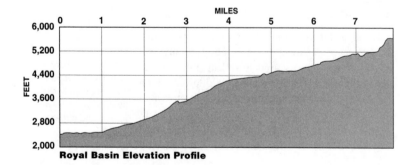

Royal Basin Elevation Profile

but remains gentle and mostly level for the first mile to a junction ▶2 just before a log bridge spanning the cascading and slightly milky waters of Royal Creek.

You go right at the junction (do *not* cross the bridge), make two short switchbacks, and soon come to a signed junction with Lower Maynard Burn Trail, which goes sharply right. Keep straight on the main trail and begin a long, steady, but never overly steep climb. Not quite 0.3 mile after the Lower Maynard Burn junction, you enter Olympic National Park, where a sign reminds you that pets are no longer allowed on the trail. You keep climbing, crossing a few small and unnamed side creeks as the canyon gradually curves to the southwest. You gain your first views at about 2.7 miles when you cross a brushy and rocky avalanche chute. From here, you'll have a decent look directly up the canyon to the snowy crags of Mount Clark and Mount Walkinshaw.

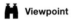

You pass a very nice campsite ▶3 beside Royal Creek about 0.1 mile after this first viewpoint. About 1.5 miles later, after a noticeably steeper section and two switchbacks, you come to another avalanche chute and a fine viewpoint ▶4 of Mount Clark directly in front of you.

At 6.3 miles, the trail levels out and crosses a willow-choked subalpine meadow, where a sign directs you to the Lower Meadow Campsites ▶5 on your right. In the latter half of July, this meadow supports colorful displays of lupine, buttercup, bistort, valerian, and other wildflowers. Just more than 100 yards past the turnoff to the Lower Meadow Campsites, you come to a log bridge over Royal Creek. A final uphill with five switchbacks leads you to the north shore of Royal Lake. ▶6 This small but extremely scenic gem is hemmed in by 7,000-foot peaks, including Mount Clark and Mount Deception, so be sure to take some time to explore its shores and admire the views. A pleasant and very scenic trail goes around the lake. Several very good campsites

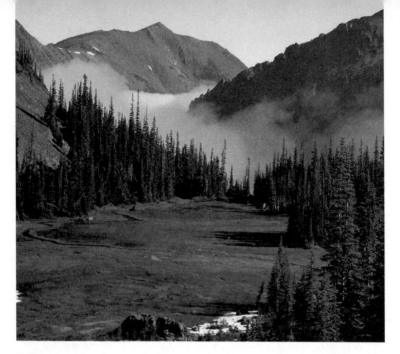

Baldy *over meadow above Royal Lake*

are hidden amid the trees and hummocks west of the lake. Remember that all overnight stays require a reserved, limited-use camping permit and that you are only allowed to camp at specific designated sites.

Day hikers can turn around here, feeling well compensated for their efforts by the beauty of aptly named Royal Lake. Backpackers, however, will have the time for some additional wildly scenic exploring. By far, the best option is to take the trail that goes past several campsites on the west side of Royal Lake to a flat meadow with excellent views of extremely rugged Mount Clark. Near the edge of this meadow is a turnoff to the former site of a seasonal ranger's tent. Just beyond this turnoff is a junction. Keep right, following a sign to Upper Basin, and take a steep, irregularly maintained trail that leads up to a lush, flat upper meadow.

Steep

At the south end of this meadow, you rock-hop what's left of Royal Creek below a crashing waterfall, and then go up a gully that is often filled with snow

Waterfall

for much of the summer. At the top, you reach the rolling alpine paradise of Upper Royal Basin. Nearly surrounded by 7,000-foot peaks, this is one of the scenic wonders of Olympic National Park. In late July, the boggy alpine meadows in the upper basin are home to a wealth of beautiful, water-loving wildflowers, especially elephant's-heads, alpine buttercups, shooting stars, and marsh marigolds. You can explore this wonderland to your heart's content. Of particular interest is a small pond ▶7 off to your right (west) that features great views and reflections of the nearby snowy peaks. Once you've seen enough (which could take a while), return the way you came, probably smiling all the way back to the trailhead. ▶8

 Wildflowers

 Lake

🚶	**MILESTONES**	
▶1	0.0	Dungeness Trailhead parking lot (N47° 52.651' W123° 08.221')
▶2	1.0	Junction with Royal Basin Trail (N47° 52.148' W123° 09.044')
▶3	2.8	Creek-side campsite (N47° 52.279' W123° 11.199')
▶4	4.3	Second viewpoint (N47° 51.383' W123° 12.683')
▶5	6.3	Lower Meadow Campsite (N47° 50.345' W123° 12.680')
▶6	7.0	Royal Lake (N47° 49.976' W123° 12.678')
▶7	7.9	Pond in Upper Royal Basin (N47° 49.315' W123° 13.146')
▶8	15.8	Return to trailhead (N47° 52.651' W123° 08.221')

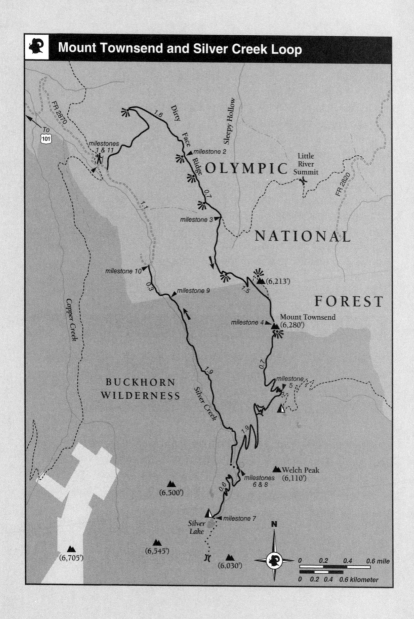

FR 2870

To
101

milestones
1 & 11

Dirty Face Ridge

1.6

milestone 2

Sleepy Hollow

OLYMPIC

Little
River
Summit

FR 2820

0.7

milestone 3

NATIONAL

milestone 10

0.3

milestone 9

1.5

(6,213')

FOREST

1.1

Copper Creek

BUCKHORN
WILDERNESS

Silver Creek

1.9

milestone 4

Mount Townsend
(6,280')

0.7

milestone
5

1.9

Welch Peak
(6,110')

milestones
6 & 8

0.6

(6,500')

Silver
Lake

milestone 7

N

(6,705')

(6,545')

(6,030')

0   0.2   0.4   0.6 mile

0   0.2   0.4   0.6 kilometer

Mount Townsend and Silver Creek Loop

Several hundred (possibly even thousands) of people trek to the top of Mount Townsend every year, numbers that are explained by the fact that this lofty peak provides one of the finest views in the eastern Olympics. Though this is perfectly reasonable (the view really is stupendous), in my opinion virtually all of these people do it the wrong way. More than 95% of hikers approach the mountain on one of two trails coming from the east. And while those are nice trails and make for good hikes, they really don't compare on the scenery scale with the route from the north along view-packed Dirty Face Ridge. True, the trailhead is a little harder to reach and the trail itself is very steep in places, but if its scenery you desire, then the Dirty Face Ridge route is definitely for you.

The backpacker, or really athletic and ambitious day hiker, can turn this into a long and challenging loop trip that visits a lovely little cirque lake tucked beneath a snowy ridge (nice camps) and then returns to the trailhead via Silver Lake Way Trail. Although this unofficial path is unsigned, steep, and rugged, it is nonetheless reasonably easy to follow and makes a good shortcut back to the starting point for experienced hikers.

Best Time

The trail is usually open June–October. Mid- to late June is ideal for alpine wildflowers as well as for providing the best photo opportunities because the peaks are still streaked with snow. Definitely save this for a clear day, and be sure to get an early start,

TRAIL USE
Day hiking, backpacking, dogs allowed

LENGTH
7.6 miles, 4–5 hours (for Mount Townsend); 10.9 miles, 6 hours or 2 days (for loop)

CUMULATIVE ELEVATION
3,100' (to Mount Townsend); 4,000' (loop)

DIFFICULTY
- 1 2 3 4 **5** +

TRAIL TYPE
Out-and-back (to Mount Townsend); Loop (for Silver Creek Loop)

SURFACE TYPE
Dirt

CONTOUR MAP
Green Trails *Tyler Peak* #136 or Custom Correct *Buckhorn Wilderness*

START & END
N47° 53.174'
W123° 05.495'

FEATURES
Dramatic 360-degree views over most of the Olympic Mountains and across Puget Sound, mountain lake

FACILITIES
None

so you can tackle the steep climb up Dirty Face Ridge in the cool and shade of the morning.

Finding the Trail

Leave US 101 about 1.5 miles east of Sequim near milepost 267.2 at a junction just southeast of the turnoff for John Wayne Marina. Turn south on Palo Alto Road and follow this good, paved, county road for 8.3 miles to a road fork, where signs point right to Dungeness Forks Campground. Bear right (downhill) on gravel Forest Road 2880 and drive 1.7 miles on this narrow road to a prominent junction with FR 2870. Go left here, following signs to Dungeness Trail, and proceed 2.6 miles to another major junction. Keep right, still on FR 2870, and drive 6.6 miles to the large Dungeness Trailhead parking area on the right just after a bridge over the Dungeness River. Continue driving on FR 2870 for another 3.8 miles and then pull into the signed Tubal Cain Trailhead on the right side of the road.

Trail Description

To find the trail, walk about 200 yards farther along FR 2870 as it continues uphill from the Tubal Cain Trailhead, ▶1 and then leave that vehicle route for

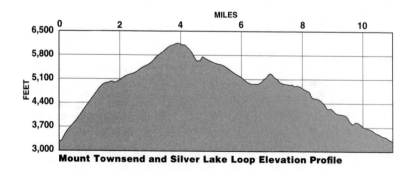

Mount Townsend and Silver Lake Loop Elevation Profile

an obvious foot trail that goes up the rocky bank on the left (northeast) side of the road. A small brown sign here identifies this as Little Quilcene Trail #835.

The path has a lot of climbing to do, and it gets right down to business. You charge up the slope at a very steep angle through forest and thickets of late-June-blooming rhododendrons. The steep and tiring uphill continues unabated, but you are compensated with lots of bright pink rhododendron blossoms and frequent partial views of numerous impressive peaks, including Buckhorn Mountain, Baldy, The Needles, Gray Wolf Ridge, and Tyler Peak. Those views only improve as you gain elevation.

Steep

Wildflowers

Viewpoint

You reach a rounded switchback at about 0.9 mile, from which you'll catch your first look at the top of Mount Townsend to the south–southeast. At just shy of 1.6 miles, and after gaining a ridiculous 1,850 feet, you reach the top of Dirty Face Ridge. ►2 At this point, two very good things happen: The pace of your climb slackens noticeably, and terrific unimpeded views open up to the west and southwest. From here, you can see much of the upper drainages of Dungeness River, Royal Creek, Copper Creek, and Silver Creek, as well as the countless snowy peaks that enclose and divide those streams. It's a wonderful vista, and the trip is not over yet!

Viewpoint

The now up-and-down trail goes south–southeast, generally at or near the top of Dirty Face Ridge. The tree cover is relatively sparse here with ground-hugging junipers, subalpine firs, and scraggly lodgepole pines being the dominant species. You pass numerous impressive basalt rock outcrops along the way and enjoy almost continuous views either west to the Olympic Mountains, east to the Puget Sound lowlands and the distant Cascade Range, or north to the Strait of Juan de Fuca. At 2.3 miles is a junction. ►3 This is one of the two much

Geologic Interest

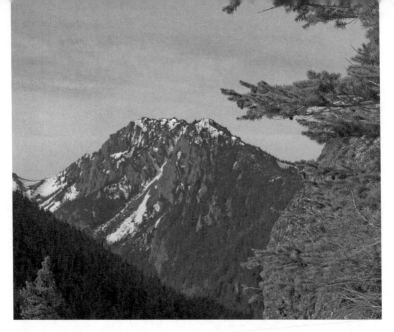

Unnamed peak *southwest of Dirty Face Ridge*

more popular trails to Mount Townsend, so you can expect company from here to the top.

Keep right at the junction and begin a steady, moderately graded ascent, still generally staying near the top of Dirty Face Ridge, which now becomes the northern approach ridge to Mount Townsend. The views are hidden for about 0.2 mile, but then they return with gusto, especially the vistas of the jagged group of peaks clustered around Buckhorn Mountain to the southwest. About halfway up this latest climb, you enter the Buckhorn Wilderness, after which the terrain becomes increasingly open and alpine in character with fewer (and much shorter) trees. After two switchbacks, you come to an unsigned junction.

Viewpoint 🔭

The trail that switchbacks to the left is an unofficial path that climbs steeply to the north summit of Mount Townsend before looping back to the main trail. The official trail goes straight at the junction and climbs gradually to a wide, treeless saddle where it rejoins the trail from the north summit. From there, you continue south over open view-packed slopes to the southern and higher summit of Mount Townsend. ▶4 The views here extend over large parts of the Olympic Mountains as well as north to Vancouver Island and east to the many arms of Puget Sound and the rugged Cascade Range. The tall, pointed mountain now visible to the south–southwest is Mount Constance.

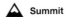 **Summit**

 Viewpoint

After at least an hour or so to enjoy the view, most day hikers should turn around here, more than satisfied with the compensation for their efforts. Backpackers and very athletic day hikers, however, have additional options. For overnight hikers, the easiest alternative (but *only* if the weather is good) is to find a flat and rocky spot (*not* on the fragile tundra vegetation, please) near the summit and set up your tent. You can usually rely on lingering snowfields for water, at least until about early July. *Tip:* Be sure to wander to the summit a little before sunset to enjoy a magnificent color show as the sun goes down over the Olympic Mountains to the west.

Another option is Silver Lake and the rugged loop back along Silver Creek. To reach that goal, continue straight on the heavily used trail down the south side of Mount Townsend. This well-graded route descends 10 switchbacks initially over tundra and then across mostly open slopes with scattered trees. At 0.7 mile from the top is a junction. ▶5

The most popular approach trail to Mount Townsend goes left here, but you turn right on the lesser-used route to Silver Lake. Over the next 0.3 mile, this trail ascends four short switchbacks to a notch in the ridge. From here, you have excellent views to the west over the entire Silver Creek drainage.

 Viewpoint

The scenic trail now goes down the sometimes rocky west side of the ridge, descending toward Silver Creek, which you can hear in the valley below you. The gently graded trail employs five long switchbacks to take you down to a large spring a little above Silver Creek. ►6 Although there is no sign, this is the start of Silver Lake Way Trail, the rough but reasonably good possible return trail for the loop.

Before taking that route, however, you won't want to miss the side trip to scenic Silver Lake. So stick with the main trail that goes south from the spring and wind your way uphill for 0.6 mile, gaining about 400 feet along the way, to the north shore and outlet of fairly small Silver Lake. ►7 The lake basin is tucked into the north side of a high ridge, and it remains snowbound until at least late June. Once the white stuff is gone, however, you will find a couple of excellent campsites near the lake's outlet with fine views of the nearby peaks. If you are up for some exploring, consider scrambling up the ridge to the south to an obvious pass and its vistas.

Lake 〰

If you are a novice hiker or are navigationally challenged (please, be honest with yourself when making this assessment), then you should return to your car on the same well-marked trail over Mount Townsend that you came in on. But if you possess halfway decent hiking and navigation skills, it is fairly simple to take Silver Lake Way Trail for a shorter return route to your car. To find it, return to the spring ►8 about 0.6 mile below Silver Lake and look for orange flags tied to tree limbs on the south side of the creek that flows from the spring. Turn onto this route and after less than 20 yards, you'll notice that the tread becomes fairly obvious. The unofficial route is "maintained" (to a minimal standard) by a local hiking club and remains reasonably easy to follow throughout its length. The club members have even installed orange flags at the handful of confusing places and cut some logs across the path as needed.

Steep

The often rugged and occasionally steep and slippery route (watch your footing) follows the left (west) side of Silver Creek on a little ridge for about

0.2 mile, and then crosses the stream and remains faithful to the right (east) side most of the rest of the way down. After 1.9 miles, you reach the unsigned wilderness boundary and emerge at the upper (south) end of an old clear-cut. ▸9 A sharp little downhill then takes you to a plank crossing of the creek and a short section of steep little ups and downs on the opposite bank. This leads to a long abandoned and overgrown dirt road (now just a wide trail) that you follow for 0.15 mile to an unofficial trailhead at a curve in gravel FR 2870. ▸10 Go right here and walk mostly downhill along this road for 1.1 miles back to the Tubal Cain Trailhead. ▸11

大	MILESTONES	
▸1	0.0	Start at Tubal Cain Trailhead (N47° 53.174' W123° 05.495')
▸2	1.6	Top of Dirty Face Ridge (N47° 53.288' W123° 04.568')
▸3	2.3	Junction (N47° 52.829' W123° 04.156')
▸4	3.8	Summit of Mount Townsend (N47° 52.046' W123° 03.571')
▸5	4.5	Junction (N47° 51.550' W123° 03.531')
▸6	6.4	Spring above Silver Creek (N47° 51.041' W123° 03.974')
▸7	7.0	Silver Lake (N47° 50.691' W123° 04.237')
▸8	7.6	Back to spring and start of Silver Lake Way Trail (N47° 51.041' W123° 03.974')
▸9	9.5	Upper edge of old clear-cut (N47° 52.284' W123° 04.778')
▸10	9.8	Gravel Forest Road 2870 (N47° 52.468' W123° 04.940')
▸11	10.9	Return to trailhead (N47° 53.174' W123° 05.495')

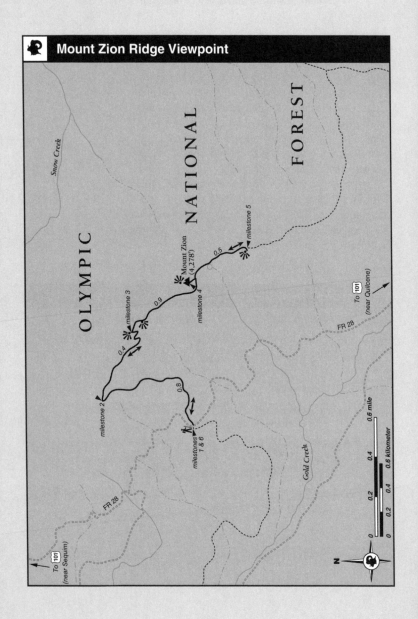

Mount Zion Ridge Viewpoint

OLYMPIC

NATIONAL

FOREST

Snow Creek

milestone 5

Mount Zion
(4,278')

0.5

milestone 3

0.9

milestone 4

0.4

milestone 2

0.8

milestones
1 & 6

Gold Creek

FR 28

To 101
(near Quilcene)

To 101
(near Sequim)

FR 28

N

0   0.2   0.4   0.6 kilometer

0   0.2   0.4   0.6 mile

Mount Zion Ridge Viewpoint

Mount Zion is an isolated peak far from the more popular trails on national park land, but it offers national park–caliber scenery. Though the old fire lookout building at the summit is long gone and trees now block most of the view, savvy hikers know that all is not lost and the former views are still available. By continuing your hike less than 0.5 mile beyond the summit, you come to a superb rocky overlook with unobstructed vistas that extend across a wide range of rugged peaks and forested valleys. If you time your hike for the latter part of June, you can enjoy acres of pink-blooming rhododendrons along the climb to the top. It's a terrific one-two punch from such a relatively short hike.

Best Time

The trail is usually hikable May–late October. Mid- to late June is ideal for blooming rhododendrons, and clear skies are needed to fully savor the views.

Finding the Trail

There are two ways to drive to the trailhead. Unfortunately, neither route is particularly well signed, and both are often confusing because the road numbers on the signs have been changed and don't always match those shown on some US Forest Service maps. Even the US Forest Service's own literature is contradictory, with some sources saying the trailhead is on Forest Road 28, others indicating that it is on FR 2849, and the US Forest Service

TRAIL USE
Day hiking, mountain biking, horses, dogs allowed, child-friendly, motorcycles allowed (but rare)

LENGTH
4.6 miles, 3 hours

CUMULATIVE ELEVATION
1,450'

DIFFICULTY
- 1 2 **3** 4 5 +

TRAIL TYPE
Out-and-back

SURFACE TYPE
Dirt

CONTOUR MAP
Custom Correct *Buckhorn Wilderness* or Green Trails *Tyler Peak* #136

START & END
N47° 55.374'
W123° 01.567'

FEATURES
Excellent views, abundant rhododendrons

FACILITIES
Restrooms, picnic table

275

map showing that it is on FR 2810. (According to the rangers, the *correct* number should be FR 28, and they are trying to change all the relevant signs to reflect this.) Watch your odometer and carefully follow the directions below so you don't get lost.

The slightly easier drive is from the east. To use this approach, leave US 101 a little less than 2 miles north of Quilcene near milepost 292.7, where you turn west on Lords Lake Loop Road. Drive this paved road for 3.4 miles to a junction beside Lords Lake (a dammed reservoir). You go left here, drive 0.7 mile, and then keep right at a lesser (and probably unsigned) junction. Keep right this time, now on gravel FR 28, and proceed 3.5 miles to a junction with FR 27. Bear right, still on FR 28, and drive 1.3 miles to a junction at Bon Jon Pass. Go right, still on FR 28 (though the signs here may not agree), and drive a final 2.1 miles to the trailhead.

A more direct route for hikers coming from the north is to leave US 101 about 1.5 miles east of Sequim near milepost 267.2 at a junction just southeast of the turnoff for John Wayne Marina. Turn south on Palo Alto Road and follow this good, paved, county road for 8.3 miles to a road fork, where signs point right to Dungeness Forks Campground. You keep straight (slightly left) and reach

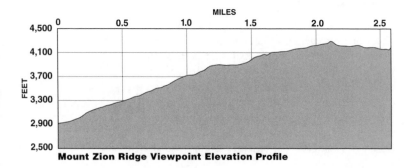

Mount Zion Ridge Viewpoint Elevation Profile

the end of pavement 0.3 mile later, where a gravel US Forest Service road angles in from the left. Keep straight, on what is signed as FR 28 (your map may not agree), and proceed 3.7 miles to an unsigned fork. Go right, and after another 1.5 miles come to a second fork. Keep left on the main road, drive 1 mile, keep left at yet another fork, and go a final 1.3 miles to the large trailhead parking area on the right.

Trail Description

The signed Mount Zion Trail begins on the opposite side of the road from the trailhead parking lot. ►1 The path wastes no time with warm-ups, as it immediately begins climbing through a forest dominated by Douglas-firs and western hemlocks. The forest here is notably drier than what you find on the west side of the range, without the rain forest's hanging mosses or abundant lichens. What is abundant here, however, is Washington's state flower, the Pacific rhododendron. These broadleaf evergreen shrubs cannot survive the drowning that plants must endure on the west side of the peninsula, but they thrive here in the marginally drier rain shadow of the range. In fact, there are few better places in the state to appreciate this plant than the slopes of Mount Zion, where from time to time you will walk through virtual tunnels of 15-foot-high flowering shrubs. Needless to say, the displays of pink blossoms in mid- to late June are breathtaking.

 Wildflowers

Also breathtaking (literally) is the climb, which is steady and moderately steep. The wide trail soon curves to the left and makes an extended uphill traverse, always in the shade of trees. Along the way, you'll cross a couple of gullies that sometimes have trickles of water in them, though, as always, you are better off carrying your own water.

 Steep

At about 0.8 mile, you come to a rounded switchback. ►2 Increasing numbers of small openings in

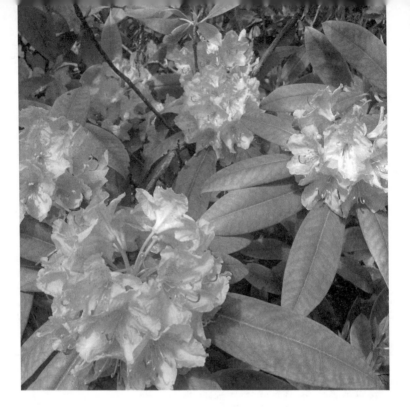

Blooming *Pacific rhododendrons*

the forest provide peekaboo looks at distant craggy mountains but not yet the full panorama that you would like. After another 0.3 mile, you come to a series of short switchbacks. At the fourth and final switchback, an obvious scramble path goes straight and in just 20 yards takes you to a rocky overlook ▶3 with excellent views of Mount Townsend to the south and a host of jagged ridges to the southwest.

Viewpoint

The main trail makes a sharp right turn at the switchback and 100 yards later passes a second fine viewpoint just below the trail on the right. Two more uphill switchbacks and an extended traverse just below a ridgeline finally leads to the rocky summit of Mount Zion. ▶4 The foundations of the fire lookout that once stood here are gone, but there are still good views to the north and east over Puget

Summit

Sound to the Cascade Mountains. Unfortunately, young trees now block the views to the south and west. Correcting this problem requires a bit more work, but it is well worth it.

Follow the trail that continues along the forested ridge going south–southeast and soon pass a small spring that used to provide water for the fire lookout. The ridge then does a bit of up and down but never gains or loses too much elevation. At not quite 0.5 mile from the summit, you reach the base of a large rocky outcrop on your right. Unless you are severely acrophobic, it's relatively easy to scramble to the top of this dramatic ridgetop overlook, ▶5 where you are treated to superb views of Mount Townsend, Tyler Peak, The Needles, and countless other snowy ridges and peaks in the Olympic Mountains. Savor the scene for as long as you like, and then return to the trailhead ▶6 the way you came.

 Viewpoint

<table>
<tr><td colspan="3">🚶   **MILESTONES**</td></tr>
<tr><td>▶1</td><td>0.0</td><td>Take trail from parking lot (N47° 55.374' W123° 01.567')</td></tr>
<tr><td>▶2</td><td>0.8</td><td>Rounded switchback (N47° 55.768' W123° 01.416')</td></tr>
<tr><td>▶3</td><td>1.2</td><td>Rocky overlook (N47° 55.606' W123° 00.930')</td></tr>
<tr><td>▶4</td><td>2.1</td><td>Summit of Mount Zion (N47° 55.402' W123° 00.637')</td></tr>
<tr><td>▶5</td><td>2.6</td><td>Ridge viewpoint (N47° 55.092' W124° 00.397')</td></tr>
<tr><td>▶6</td><td>5.2</td><td>Return to trailhead (N47° 55.374' W123° 01.567')</td></tr>
</table>

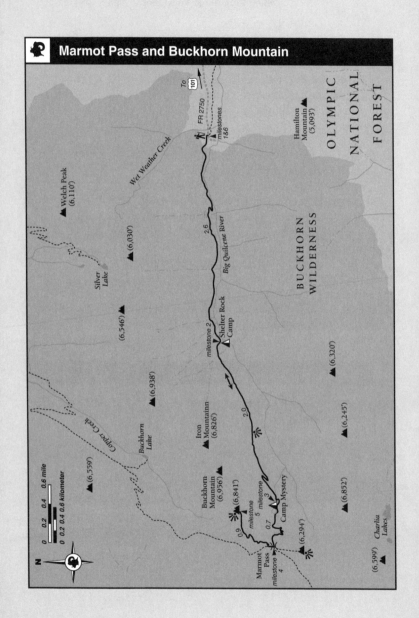

Marmot Pass and Buckhorn Mountain

Welch Peak
(6,110) ▲

(6,030) ▲

Silver Lake

(6,546) ▲

Wet Weather Creek

To 101

FR 2750

milestones 1 & 6

Hamilton Mountain (5,093') ▲

OLYMPIC   NATIONAL   FOREST

BUCKHORN   WILDERNESS

Big Quilcene River

2.6

milestone 2

Shelter Rock Camp

(6,320') ▲

2.0

(6,245') ▲

(6,938') ▲

Iron Mountainn (6,826') ▲

Buckhorn Lake

Copper Creek

(6,559') ▲

Buckhorn Mountain (6,956') ▲

(6,841') ▲

0.9   milestone 3

milestone 5   0.7   Camp Mystery

(6,294') ▲

(6,852') ▲

Charlia Lakes

(6,599') ▲

Marmot Pass   milestone 4

N

0   0.2   0.4   0.6 mile
0   0.2 0.4 0.6 kilometer

Marmot Pass and Buckhorn Mountain

This is a very popular trail that was once described in another guidebook as being the best day hike on the Olympic Peninsula. I think that is an overstatement, but there is no denying that this is a wonderful hike with a great deal of variety along the way. Here, you will enjoy miles of ancient forests, a clear and cascading stream, plenty of wildflowers, the opportunity to see wildlife, and stupendous views from trail's end. Though better examples of all of these features can be found on other trips, few hikes can boast of including them all on the same trail. The journey is relatively long, so only fairly strong day hikers should attempt it, but it can also be done as a moderate overnight hike, which would allow you to stay longer and enjoy the trip's many charms.

Best Time

The trail is usually open July–October. Wildflowers peak in July. Save this hike for a clear day, to wholly appreciate the views. Start early in the morning because the trip is fairly long, and the cool of the morning is more comfortable during the climb.

Finding the Trail

Leave US 101 about 1.5 miles south of Quilcene near milepost 296.2. Turn west here onto Penny Creek Road and drive this paved route for 1.5 miles to a prominent fork. Go left on gravel County Road 3057, following signs to Big Quilcene and Mount Townsend Trails, and proceed 2 miles to another fork. Go right, back onto a one-lane paved road that

TRAIL USE
Day hiking, backpacking, horses (though rare), dogs allowed

LENGTH
10.6 miles, 5–6 hours or 2 days (for Marmot Pass); 12.4 miles, 7–8 hours or 2 days (for Buckhorn Mountain)

CUMULATIVE ELEVATION
3,650' (to Marmot Pass); 4,640' (to Buckhorn Mountain)

DIFFICULTY
- 1 2 3 4 **5** +

TRAIL TYPE
Out-and-back

SURFACE TYPE
Dirt

CONTOUR MAP
Green Trails *Tyler Peak* #136 or Custom Correct *Buckhorn Wilderness*

START & END
N47° 49.665'
W123° 02.470'

FEATURES
Clear and tumbling stream, lots of wildflowers, wildlife, alpine views

FACILITIES
Restrooms

281

now becomes Forest Road 27, and drive 1.2 miles to a junction. Go right, still on paved FR 27, and continue 6.3 miles to another junction. Turn left (west) onto FR 2750, following signs to Big Quilcene Trail, and drive this gravel road 4.9 miles to the trailhead. Parking is on the left (south) side of the road.

Trail Description

Take the Upper Big Quilcene Trail, which leaves from the north side of the gravel road across from the trailhead parking area ▶1.

Old-Growth Forest

The wide trail begins in old-growth forest (as do so many trails in the Olympics), almost immediately enters the Buckhorn Wilderness, and gradually traverses a hillside above the tumbling waters of the initially unseen Big Quilcene River. The trail soon gets close to the creek (calling it a river at this point is overly generous) and closely follows this clear stream for the next 1.4 miles. At this point, two quick switchbacks take you up onto the hillside to the north and to a crossing of a small tributary creek

Waterfall

just below a lacy little waterfall. From here, you continue west, climbing a series of steep sections that are interspersed with places where the route is

Steep

quite gentle. After crossing several small creeks, you come to Shelter Rock Camp ▶2 at 2.6 miles. Here,

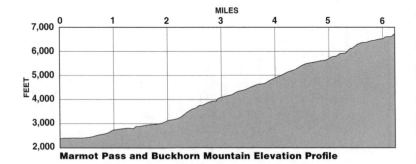

Marmot Pass and Buckhorn Mountain Elevation Profile

there is a large flat area just to the left of the trail that can accommodate numerous tents. Despite the name, there is no large (or, for that matter, small) sheltering rock nearby.

Still in attractive forest, the trail climbs steadily away from the "river" onto a hillside where the forest gradually becomes more open. This allows occasional views of a dark, craggy ridge to the southwest with several jagged pinnacles and sheer cliffs. The scenery just gets better as you continue climbing, often over rocky slopes with an abundance of wildflowers. In **Wildflowers**
July you should expect to see Indian paintbrush, stonecrop, larkspur, Sitka valerian, woolly yellow daisy, wallflower, lupine, spreading phlox, columbine, and Lomatium, among others. While the forest opens up, it also changes its makeup, with higher-elevation species, such as Alaska yellow cedar and subalpine fir, becoming dominant.

At 4.6 miles, you reach Camp Mystery ▸3. This is a popular overnight spot because it has numerous comfortable tent sites, nice scenery, and a large spring and creek that provide the last reliable water along the trail.

For the trip's main attraction, keep climbing from Camp Mystery, at first beside a narrow, wildflower-covered meadow and then switchbacking up a partly forested slope. You top out at a signed junction at often-windy Marmot Pass. ▸4 The view **Viewpoint**
to the west from here is beyond outstanding. Rising above the deep canyon of the Dungeness River is a string of tall snow-streaked summits, including Mounts Fricaba, Mystery, Deception, Clark, and Walkinshaw. All of these peaks exceed 7,000 feet and are among the highest points in the Olympic Mountains. If you can tear your eyes off the scenery (good luck), you might also notice that the trees here are mostly stunted whitebark pines, a species that only grows in a handful of places around the  **Wildlife**
Olympic Mountains. Wildlife you may see here

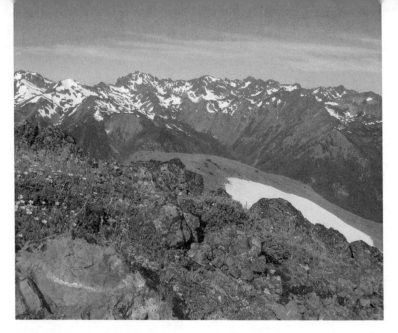

View west *from Buckhorn Mountain*

includes mountain goats, Olympic chipmunks, deer, and, of course, Olympic marmots, for whom the pass was named.

If you still have energy once you reach Marmot Pass, and a view like this tends to reenergize even the most tired hiker, expend it on some rewarding nearby exploring. The trail to the south–southwest traverses view-packed slopes for the next mile or so, offering fairly easy and very scenic hiking. Closer at hand, a boot trail leads almost due south to the top of a rounded summit immediately south of Marmot Pass that provides even wider views. In the other direction, the trail to the north crosses steep tundra and partly forested slopes with plenty of unobstructed views in all directions.

For the highest and best views of all, however, climb to the top of a rounded butte on the side of Buckhorn Mountain, the towering summit that rises to the northeast of Marmot Pass. To reach it, take the trail going north for about 110 yards to a small cairn that marks an obvious boot path going uphill to the right. Take this path and climb, very steeply at times, soon finding yourself in an above-timberline realm dominated by rocks, low-growing grasses, wildflowers, and, of course, wide views. Once you reach the top of the rounded butte, ▶5 those views encompass not only all the peaks previously listed but also Baldy to the north–northwest, Mount Constance and Warrior Peak to the south, and the distant volcanic mountains of the Cascade Range to the east. The actual summit of Buckhorn Mountain is the rugged peak about 0.25 mile to the northeast. Reaching this spot requires some tricky scrambling and mountain climbing skills. In addition, the view from the actual summit is no better than it is from the slightly lower butte, so it really isn't worth it. *Warning:* Be very careful on the way back down to Marmot Pass because it's easy to lose your footing on the steep sections with all the loose rocks and pebbles. The way back down to the trailhead ▶6 from Marmot Pass, though long, is not as steep, so it poses no such difficulties.

 Steep

 Summit

 Viewpoint

🚶	**MILESTONES**	
▶1	0.0	Trailhead (N47° 49.665' W123° 02.470')
▶2	2.6	Shelter Rock Camp (N47° 49.505' W123° 05.390')
▶3	4.6	Camp Mystery (N47° 49.048' W123° 07.439')
▶4	5.3	Marmot Pass (N47° 49.083' W123° 08.007')
▶5	6.2	Summit of butte below Buckhorn Mountain (N47° 49.392' W123° 07.530')
▶6	12.4	Return to trailhead (N47° 49.665' W123° 02.470')

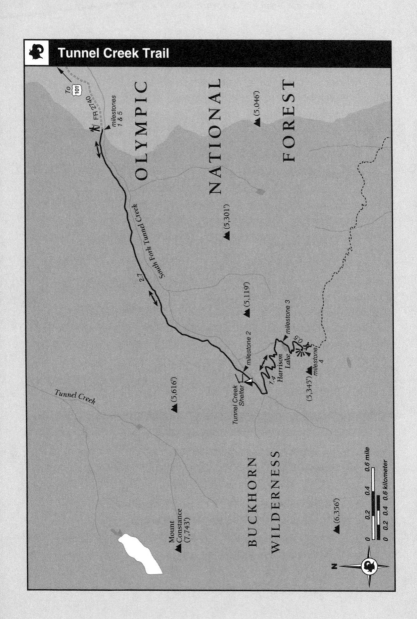

Tunnel Creek Trail

OLYMPIC   NATIONAL   FOREST

To 101

FR 2740

milestones 1 & 5

▲ (5,046')

▲ (5,301')

South Fork Tunnel Creek

2.7

▲ (5,119')

milestone 2

milestone 3

0.5

Tunnel Creek
Shelter

Harrison
Lake

1/4

milestone 4

▲ (5,616')

▲ (5,345')

Tunnel Creek

BUCKHORN

WILDERNESS

▲ (6,356')

Mount
Constance
(7,743')

N

0   0.2   0.4   0.6 mile

0   0.2   0.4 0.6 kilometer

Tunnel Creek Trail

This hike takes you through forest and along a lovely creek to an old trail shelter. Early in the season, it can be done as an enjoyable cloudy weather leg stretcher. By July, however, you can extend the hike to a subalpine lake and a high ridge that offers perhaps the peninsula's best trail-accessible viewpoint of Mount Constance, the third-highest peak in the Olympic Mountains. Either route is fun and worth doing, and you won't be disappointed to visit this trail more than once as your time and the seasons permit.

Best Time

The lower trail is typically open by May, but the upper trail to the ridge viewpoint does not open until very late June or early July. If you just want a relatively easy and fun forest walk, then any weather is fine, but if you are continuing to the ridge viewpoint, clear skies are required to fully enjoy it.

Finding the Trail

Leave US 101 about 1.5 miles south of Quilcene near milepost 296.2. Turn west here onto Penny Creek Road and drive this paved route for 1.5 miles to a prominent fork. Go left on gravel County Road 3057, following signs to Big Quilcene and Mount Townsend Trails, and proceed 2 miles to another fork. Go right, back onto a one-lane paved road that now becomes Forest Road 27, and drive 1.2 miles to a junction. Go left here onto FR 2740 and follow this narrow gravel road for 7 miles to the trailhead.

TRAIL USE
Day hiking, backpacking, dogs allowed

LENGTH
9.2 miles, 5 hours

CUMULATIVE ELEVATION
2,600'

DIFFICULTY
- 1 2 3 **4** 5 +

TRAIL TYPE
Out-and-back

SURFACE TYPE
Dirt

CONTOUR MAP
Green Trails *Tyler Peak* #136 or Custom Correct *Buckhorn Wilderness*

START & END
N47° 46.880'
W123° 03.148'

FEATURES
Attractive forest walk, small lake, views of Mount Constance

FACILITIES
None

The road beyond this point has been washed out and is now blocked off by a line of huge boulders.

Trail Description

Old-Growth Forest

Wildflowers

Historic Interest

Steep

From the trailhead, ▶1 the signed Tunnel Creek Trail ascends beneath a shady canopy of big western hemlocks, western red cedars, and Douglas-firs, never straying far from the soothing sounds of clear and cascading South Fork Tunnel Creek on your left. In early July, forest wildflowers, including queen's cup, foamflower, and bunchberry, add small white highlights to the lush green surroundings. After 2.7 viewless but fun miles of gentle up-and-down hiking (more up than down), you reach the old cedar-shake-and-log Tunnel Creek Shelter. ▶2 The trail thus far makes a pleasant forest walk that is usually open by early May. Some good camping prospects can be found at the shelter.

If you prefer dramatic mountain views, however, you must keep hiking. So after a soothing rest at the shelter, pick up the trail again and, 0.2 mile later, cross the creek on a log bridge. From there, you begin a tough and often steep climb. A total of eight switchbacks help to ease the grade, and the climb only lasts for 1.1 miles, but it still requires a rest stop or two along the way. Just before the last

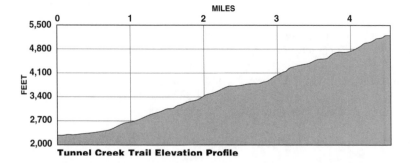
Tunnel Creek Trail Elevation Profile

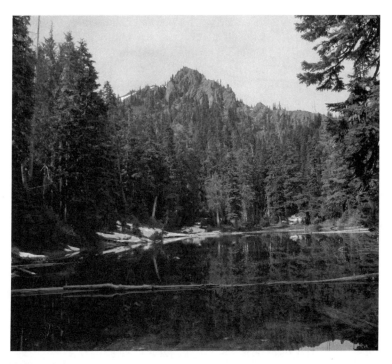

Harrison Lake

switchback, you pass a shallow pond and then complete your climb to small Harrison Lake. ▶3 There is a nice view across this shallow, pear-shaped lake to an unnamed craggy butte to the southwest.

 Lake

Though pretty, Harrison Lake still does not provide particularly dramatic scenery. To find this much sought-after feature, keep hiking the trail as it traverses the hillside on the left (southeast) side of the lake and then makes a short but fairly steep climb into a higher-elevation environment of heather, mountain hemlocks, and subalpine firs. At the top, you come to a wonderful ridgetop viewpoint ▶4 with a rocky area on your right that is ideal for sitting, eating lunch, and appreciating

 Viewpoint

the scenery. The view is dominated by the snow-streaked ramparts of the towering dark mass of Mount Constance to the northwest. At 7,743 feet, this is one of the highest peaks in the Olympic Mountains, and it is quite a sight. Other surrounding peaks, ridges, and canyons add to the scene, but Constance steals the show. Once you've had your fill, return to the trailhead ▶5 the way you came.

Note: Judged strictly by mileage, there is actually a shorter way to reach this ridgetop viewpoint that starts from a trailhead on Dosewallips River Road to the southeast. That trail is so *wickedly* steep, however, that anyone who willingly hikes it would make an interesting case study in abnormal psychology.

🚶 MILESTONES

▶1	0.0	Start at road-end trailhead (N47° 46.880' W123° 03.148')
▶2	2.7	Tunnel Creek Shelter (N47° 45.793' W123° 05.784')
▶3	4.1	Harrison Lake (N47° 45.550' W123° 05.431')
▶4	4.6	Ridge viewpoint (N47° 45.422' W123° 05.462')
▶5	9.2	Return to trailhead (N47° 46.880' W123° 03.148')

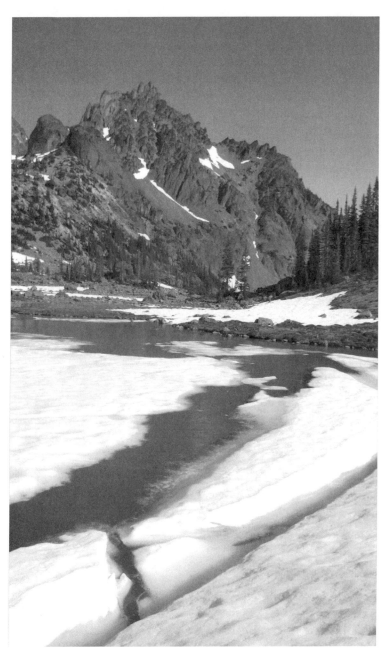

Mount Clark *over icy pond in upper Royal Basin (see Trail 31)*

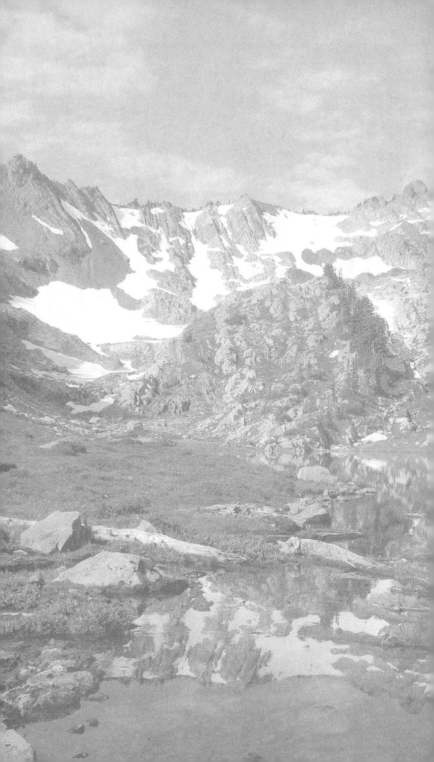

CHAPTER 6

Southeast Region: Duckabush and Skokomish Areas

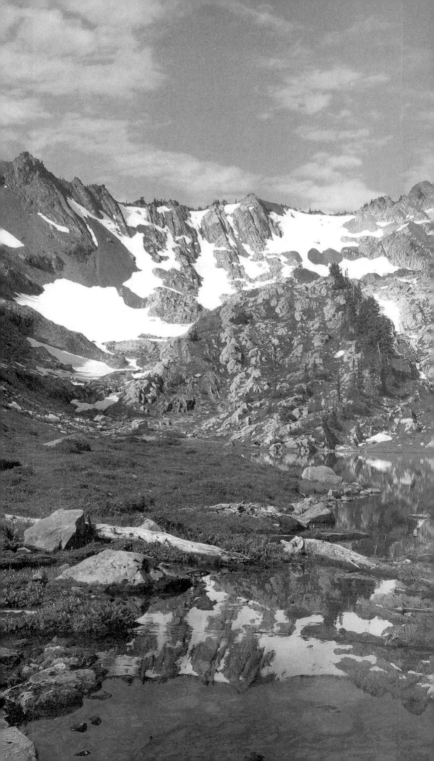

Southeast Region: Duckabush and Skokomish Areas

The relatively small southeast region is the most easily accessed by hikers who live in the heavily populated South Sound (the cities of Olympia, Tacoma, and the surrounding areas). As a result, some of the trails here are among the most heavily traveled of any on the peninsula. As often happens, however, hikers tend to congregate around a handful of traditional favorites (in particular Mount Ellinor, Flapjack Lakes, and Lena Lake), leaving the rest of the area's trails relatively lonely.

There are somewhat fewer trails in this compact area than in the other regions covered in this book, but that lack of quantity does not imply a lack of quality. The views from atop Mount Ellinor, for example, are surpassed by only a couple of places on the entire peninsula. The forests along the Staircase Rapids Trail are so lush that they come close to rivaling the much more famous rain forests along the Hoh and Quinault Rivers. Tiny Lake of the Angels may be the most beautiful trail-accessible lake on the entire peninsula. And the little-known new trail to Murhut Falls offers a fairly easy path to arguably the most impressive combination of gravity and water in the area.

The region is dominated by two large river drainages: the Duckabush to the north and the Skokomish to the south. In between is the smaller Hamma Hamma River and numerous heavily forested and steep-sided ridges. The mountains here average a little shorter than in other parts of the peninsula, so there is somewhat less alpine country to enjoy, but what does exist is dramatically scenic and well worth exploring.

The weather in this region is often wet, and it's certainly not as dry as in the Rain Shadow region to the north, but it is still noticeably drier than the country to the west, which is a blessing for those who don't much care for

Overleaf and opposite: *Lake of the Angels (Trail 37)*

hiking in the rain. As usual, the lowest elevation trails are typically hikable (and, surprisingly, not all that muddy) even in the winter, while the high country does not melt out until late June or July.

Governing Agencies

The trails to Ranger Hole and Murhut Falls (Trail 36), Mount Ellinor (Trail 38), and the lower reaches of the Lake of the Angels Trail (Trail 37) are administered by the Hood Canal Ranger District of Olympic National Forest. The Staircase Rapids (Trail 39) hike as well as the upper part of the Lake of the Angels hike is under the jurisdiction of Olympic National Park.

TRAIL FEATURES TABLE

Southeast Region: Duckabush and Skokomish Areas

TRAIL	DIFFICULTY	LENGTH	TYPE	USES & ACCESS	TERRAIN	FLORA & FAUNA	OTHER
36	2	3.4	↗	🚶 🐕 👫	🏞️ 📖		✦ 🏠
37	5	7.4	↗	🚶 🏔️	🏞️ 🌊 📖	🦌	🏠
38	4	3.4	↗	🚶 🐕	🔺 🏞️	🦌	⋈
39	1	1.8	↗	🚶 👫	📖	🌳	⋈

USES & ACCESS	TYPE	TERRAIN	FLORA & FAUNA	OTHER
🚶 Day Hiking	↻ Loop	🔺 Summit	🌳 Old-Growth Forest	⋈ Viewpoint
🏔️ Backpacking	↱ Semi-loop	🏞️ Steep		✦ Geologic Interest
🚴 Mountain Biking	↗ Out-and-back	🌊 Lake	🌸 Wildflowers	🏠 Historic Interest
🐎 Horses		📖 Waterfall	🦅 Birds	
🐕 Dogs Allowed	DIFFICULTY	✳ Tidepool	🦌 Wildlife	
👫 Child-Friendly	- 1 2 3 4 5 + less more			

Southeast Region: Duckabush and Skokomish Areas

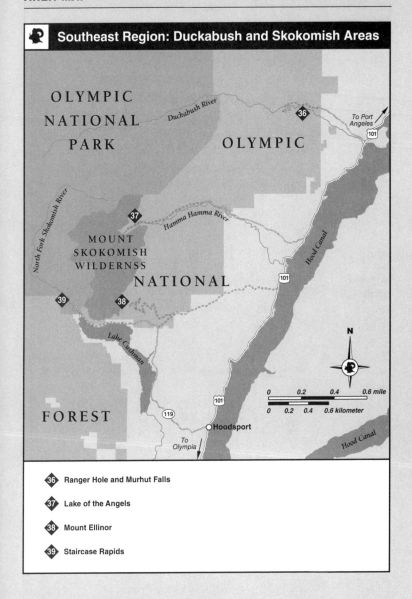

36 Ranger Hole and Murhut Falls

37 Lake of the Angels

38 Mount Ellinor

39 Staircase Rapids

Southeast Region:
Duckabush and Skokomish Areas

Ranger Hole and Murhut Falls 300

This trip combines two short and easy nearby hikes that, together, make for a very pleasant half day of hiking. The first trail descends from a historic ranger cabin to an impressive rocky canyon and fishing hole on a large river. The second trail climbs on a relatively new trail up a forested hillside to one of the most beautiful trail-accessible waterfalls on the peninsula.

Lake of the Angels 305

A ranger's favorite and arguably the prettiest trail-accessible lake in the Olympic Mountains, Lake of the Angels is incredibly beautiful. And it sure as heck better be! The "trail" here is sadistically steep and is even dangerous in a few places, where without careful foot placement and use of your hands to help pull yourself up, it would be impossible. So be prepared for a *really* tough hike, and definitely go elsewhere if you are afraid of heights or are inexperienced. But for those physically and mentally capable of making the journey, this might be the best show on the Olympic Peninsula.

Mount Ellinor

Though not an easy climb, this extremely popular trail steeply ascends to the best viewpoint in the southeastern Olympic Mountains. While the views are grand, perhaps the most famous (or notorious) feature of this hike are the resident mountain goats. These large and unpredictable animals have traditionally come quite close to hikers and sometimes even harassed visiting humans. As a result, land managers must sometimes close the trail for safety reasons. Call ahead about the latest conditions, and please do your part to discourage the animals from getting too close.

Day hiking,
dogs allowed
3.4 miles
Out-and-back
Difficulty: 1 2 3 **4** 5

Staircase Rapids

This is an easy hike through a dense and drippy forest and is suitable for hikers of all abilities and ages. The highlights are lots of big trees and the large and rambunctious North Fork Skokomish River, which drops in a series of loud and impressive cascades and waterfalls.

Day hiking,
child-friendly
1.8 miles
Out-and-back
Difficulty: **1** 2 3 4 5

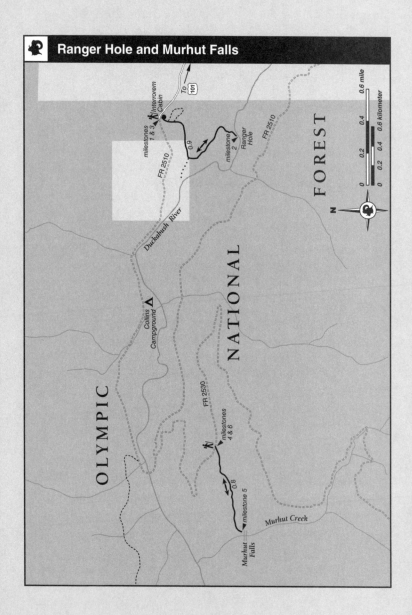

Ranger Hole and Murhut Falls

To 101

Interrorem Cabin

milestones 1 & 3

0.9

milestone 2

Ranger Hole

FR 2510

FR 2510

Duckabush River

Collins Campground

FR 2530

milestones 4 & 6

0.8

milestone 5

Murhut Falls

Murhut Creek

OLYMPIC

NATIONAL

FOREST

N

0   0.2   0.4   0.6 mile
0   0.2   0.4   0.6 kilometer

Ranger Hole and Murhut Falls

This trip combines two trails that are close to one another and short enough that you can easily hike both in an enjoyable half day. Though both routes travel through dense forest and have a water feature as their destination, the two walks are actually quite different. The Ranger Hole Trail is a historic path that wanders down to a narrow little canyon and fishing hole on the rampaging Duckabush River. The Murhut Falls route, on the other hand, was only built in the last decade or so (it isn't even on most maps yet) and travels over a ridge to one of the most impressive trail-accessible waterfalls on the Olympic Peninsula. If your time is limited and you are forced to choose, the Murhut Falls hike is somewhat more dramatic, while the Ranger Hole hike is a little easier.

Best Time

Except immediately after a rare low-elevation snowstorm, these trails are usually open all year. The scenery is best in April and May when the falls and river have high water and the new greenery is just hitting the forest. Because of the falls, these hikes are good ones to do when it's cloudy or rainy.

Finding the Trail

Leave US 101 near milepost 310, where you turn west onto County Road 2274 (also known as Duckabush Road). Follow this paved road for 3.8 miles to the boundary of Olympic National Forest, where the pavement ends and you come to the Interrorem

TRAIL USE
Day hiking, dogs allowed, child-friendly
LENGTH
3.4 miles, 2 hours (combined)
CUMULATIVE ELEVATION
570' (combined)
DIFFICULTY
- 1 **2** 3 4 5 +
TRAIL TYPE
Out-and-back
SURFACE TYPE
Dirt, gravel
CONTOUR MAP
Custom Correct *Brothers–Mt. Anderson* or Green Trails *Mt Steel* #167 (As of 2014 Murhut Falls Trail was not yet shown on these maps.)
START & END
Ranger Hole Trail:
N47° 40.882'
W122° 59.664'
Murhut Falls Trail:
N47° 40.595'
W123° 02.311'

FEATURES
Waterfall, forests, rock-lined canyon on river

FACILITIES
Hand water pump and restroom at the Ranger Hole; none at Murhut Falls

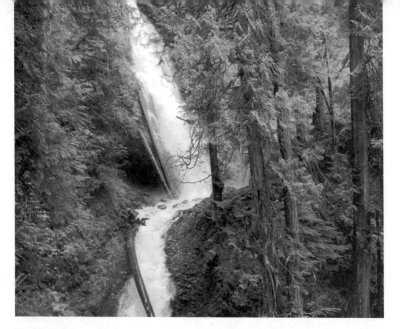

Murhut Falls

Cabin on the left. The small parking area here is the trailhead for the hike to Ranger Hole.

To find the Murhut Falls Trailhead, continue on gravel Duckabush Road (now Forest Road 2510) for another 2.6 miles to a fork just after a bridge over the Duckabush River. Go right, now on FR 2530, and proceed 1.1 miles to the Murhut Falls Trailhead on the right. There is room for about four cars to park on the left side of the road.

Trail Description

Historic Interest

Ranger Hole Trail: The signed trailhead is adjacent to a fence around the historic 1907 Interrorem Ranger Cabin. ▶1 Though rangers have not used this log building for decades, it has been beautifully restored and can now be rented out (with advance reservations) by the public to spend the night. Do not disturb those who have paid for this privilege, and please stay out of the fenced area.

The trail goes 40 yards to a pit toilet and a junction with the upper end of the short Interrorem Nature Trail Loop. Keep straight, following signs to Duckabush River, and hike a wide and gentle path that goes across a flat area with widely spaced conifers. This spacing allows in light for a particular abundance of bracken ferns, sword ferns, and vine maples—the last offering good fall color in October. Just 50 yards farther along is the second junction with the Interrorem Nature Trail Loop. Keep right and cross more of the very pretty fern-decked flat.

The partly dirt and partly gravel path remains level for the next 0.2 mile and then climbs over a low rise. From there, it descends to a prominent left turn. An abandoned and overgrown trail goes straight here, but you keep left on what is clearly the main route. The viewless trail now goes gradually downhill until the 0.7-mile point, where you reach the drop-off to the river. Here, you make a short but **Steep** steep descent before leveling out shortly before the path ends at Ranger Hole. ▶**2** At this point, Ducka- **Geologic Interest** bush River squeezes through a narrow, rocky chasm into a deep fishing hole that was once popular with the resident ranger at the Interrorem Station. A rocky overlook just above the river provides a nice view of the scene, a classic Olympic-type spot with crashing water, dense forest, and lots of surrounding greenery. Once you have enjoyed the scene, hike back to the trailhead ▶**3** the way you came.

Murhut Falls Trail: This recently completed trail climbs from the trailhead ▶**4** at a moderate grade, passing a self-registration signboard after just 80 yards. The wide and well-maintained path keeps up a steady but never steep ascent as you travel through a dense eastside Olympic Peninsula forest dominated by the big three local conifers: Douglas-firs, western hemlocks, and western red cedars. Various ferns, salal, salmonberry, twisted-stalks, trilliums, bunchberry, thimbleberry, creeping blackberry, and other understory plants crowd the forest floor.

After 0.4 mile, the trail levels out and you wander through viewless forest in little ups and downs. At 0.6 mile, after gaining about 250 feet, you reach the trail's highest point, a woodsy ridge from which you can hear the roar of the falls. A gentle downhill now takes you above a couple of smaller cascading falls to a wonderful viewpoint at trail's end ▶5 of the trip's main attraction. Thundering Murhut Falls descends in two distinct drops into a mossy canyon. With the high water and vibrant greens of spring, the falls is at its most attractive, and you will want to allow plenty of time to admire the spray-filled show. A dangerously steep scramble path goes down to the base of the falls, but it requires caution and there's not much point because the views are actually better from the main trail. So skip the exploring and simply return to the trailhead ▶6 the way you came.

Waterfall

🚶	**MILESTONES** (combined mileage)
▶1	0.0 Interrorem Ranger Station Trailhead (N47° 40.882' W122° 59.664')
▶2	0.9 Ranger Hole (N47° 40.452' W122° 59.781')
▶3	1.8 Return to Interrorem Trailhead (N47° 40.882' W122° 59.664')
▶4	1.8 Murhut Falls Trailhead (N47° 40.595' W123° 02.311')
▶5	2.6 Murhut Falls (N47° 40.460' W123° 03.001')
▶6	3.4 Return to Murhut Falls Trailhead (N47° 40.595' W123° 02.311')

Lake of the Angels

Lake of the Angels is a favorite of rangers and, arguably, the most beautiful trail-accessible lake in the Olympic Mountains. That said, in this case, the word *trail* has to be in quotes. This is one of those old boot-beaten paths so common in this range that tends to scare away all but the best conditioned and most experienced hikers. Though the route is in pretty good shape and generally easy to follow, it is also *wickedly* steep and even has a few places that are dangerously exposed, where you'll have to use your hands to both steady your nerves and help pull yourself up a steep rock face. And please keep in mind that the *downhill* on these sections is often more difficult and dangerous than going up. This is not a hike for anyone who is afraid of heights or who is unwilling to expend a lot of energy to reach the destination. So, while the rewards here are certainly great—an absolutely *stunning* little alpine lake in a setting that will draw rave reviews from even the most seasoned hiker—the costs in sweat and fear are also great and must be strongly considered before you set out from your car.

Best Time

The trail is typically open July–October. Avoid it when conditions are wet, as the steepness is hard enough without the added problems of mud and slick rocks. Late July through mid-August is ideal for flowers and the best trail conditions.

TRAIL USE
Day hiking, backpacking

LENGTH
7.4 miles, 6 hours (or overnight)

CUMULATIVE ELEVATION
3,400'

DIFFICULTY
- 1 2 3 4 **5** +

TRAIL TYPE
Out-and-back

SURFACE TYPE
Dirt

CONTOUR MAP
Custom Correct
Brothers–Mt. Anderson

START & END
N47° 47.35.005'
W123° 14.043'

FEATURES
Scenic mountain lake, exploring opportunities, tough climb

FACILITIES
None

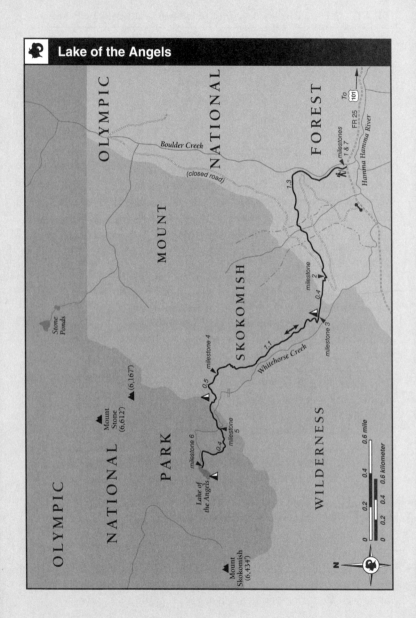

Lake of the Angels

Finding the Trail

Leave US 101 near milepost 318 and turn west on Hamma Hamma River Road, also known as Forest Road 25. Follow this good paved road for 6.5 miles to a T-junction, where you turn right, still on FR 25. Continue driving another 5.7 miles, first on pavement and then good gravel, to the signed Putvin Trailhead, immediately after a bridge over Boulder Creek.

Trail Description

The trail starts on the north side of the parking area ▶1 and heads uphill into a dense second-growth forest of western hemlocks and western red cedars. The route here is fairly steep, but this will seem absurdly easy before your day is through. At about 0.2 mile, you pass a short side trail going left to the grave of Carl Putvin, a pioneer trapper and explorer for whom this trail is named. Above this point, the trail ascends a series of steep little twists and turns past several enormous moss-covered boulders. Boulder Creek is a constant rushing companion on your right.

 Steep

Historic Interest

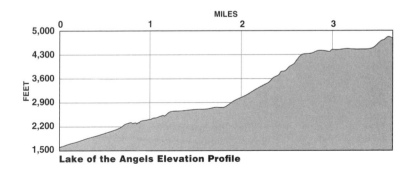
Lake of the Angels Elevation Profile

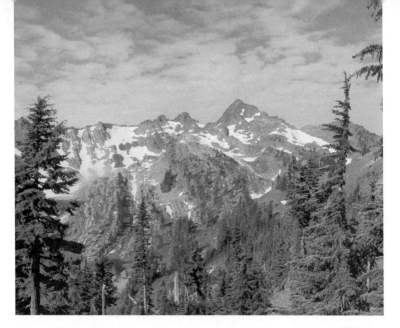

Mount Skokomish *from high route east of Lake of the Angels*

Once past the boulder field, the trail cuts to the left and makes a somewhat gentler traverse of a steep hillside. Along the way, you cross three prominent gullies. The second of these usually has water, and all three are prone to washouts. Expect to negotiate rugged little detours to get around these washouts.

At 1.3 miles, you come to an old logging road ►2 that is now largely overgrown with small trees and brush. You go left here and follow the road downhill for about 25 yards to the resumption of trail going up the hill on your right.

The route ascends six steep little switchbacks and then makes a much gentler traverse of the heavily forested hillside. A little more than 0.3 mile from the road, you pass a sign marking the boundary of the Mount Skokomish Wilderness and about 100 yards later reach a small campsite ►3 just above the trail. You can hear Whitehorse Creek cascading through the slide alder trees a little west of this camp.

Steep

Now the hard work begins as you gain some 1,600 feet in the next 1.1 miles. The trail climbs at a wickedly steep grade in little switchbacks and turns. Though steep, initially at least, the hiking through this section isn't dangerous, simply tiring. About 0.5 mile above the small campsite, you break out of the trees in an avalanche chute choked with bracken ferns, bear grass, and pearly everlasting. Not far past this, you reach the lower end of a sloping basin, choked with slide alder trees, that you can look across and glimpse waterfalls on Whitehorse Creek tumbling off a tall headwall. The top of that headwall is your goal.

 Waterfall

The rough trail climbs very steeply around the right side of this basin, eventually leading to a couple of places where you must use your hands to pull yourself up little rock chutes and over roots. Steady nerves and strong legs and lungs are required to make it up. If conditions are wet, the rock face will be slippery and even more difficult. Once this scary section is complete, you steeply ascend about another 200 feet before finally reaching the top of the headwall. ▶4

Rest here for a bit (you've earned it) before following the trail as it curves to the left (southwest) through much gentler terrain. The next 0.5 mile is delightful as the trail wanders through a mostly level basin with small ponds, lovely creeks, and pretty meadows. The route is muddy in places, but that is only a minor problem because your mind is likely preoccupied with the fact that you are no longer dealing with a steep climb. There are some nice campsites in this basin if you are willing to search for them.

You pass a sign for the boundary of Olympic National Park and just 40 yards later cross Whitehorse Creek. ▶5 A little beyond the creek crossing, the trail makes a steep, 350-foot climb on a slope covered with grasses and wildflowers. At the top of this climb is the basin holding Lake of the Angels. ▶6 Surrounded by meadows and sandwiched between towering Mount Skokomish

 Steep

 Lake

and craggy Mount Stone, this teardrop-shaped lake will take your breath away, assuming you have any breath left after that climb.

A posted map indicates the location of designated campsites that the National Park Service has established around this gem. A night spent at this lake is highly rewarding and would allow you to explore some of the very scenic ridges that surround the lake. Keep in mind, however, that to enjoy this pleasure you'll have to lug your heavy pack up that wicked trail and, often more difficult and dangerous, deal with the task of balancing this heavy pack as you make the steep downhill scramble on the return. In addition, mountain goats frequent the lake and often barge into campsites looking for handouts. A day hike is probably a better option. Return to the trailhead ▶7 on the same trail on which you came in.

 Wildlife

<table>
<tr><td colspan="3">🚶   MILESTONES</td></tr>
<tr><td>▶1</td><td>0.0</td><td>Trailhead (N47° 47.35.005' W123° 14.043')</td></tr>
<tr><td>▶2</td><td>1.3</td><td>Old logging road (N47° 35.135' W123° 14.853')</td></tr>
<tr><td>▶3</td><td>1.7</td><td>Small campsite (N47° 35.174' W123° 15.216')</td></tr>
<tr><td>▶4</td><td>2.8</td><td>Top of headwall (N47° 35.825' W123° 15.708')</td></tr>
<tr><td>▶5</td><td>3.3</td><td>Whitehorse Creek (N47° 35.737' W123° 16.090')</td></tr>
<tr><td>▶6</td><td>3.7</td><td>Lake of the Angels (N47° 35.820' W123° 16.360')</td></tr>
<tr><td>▶7</td><td>7.4</td><td>Return to trailhead (N47° 47.35.005' W123° 14.043')</td></tr>
</table>

Mount Ellinor

Without argument, Mount Ellinor offers the finest on-trail viewpoint in the southeastern Olympic Mountains. Because this portion of the range is also the most easily accessible to day hikers who live in the heavily populated Olympia and Tacoma areas, it's not surprising that this is a very popular trail. In fact, despite the trail's steep grade and considerable elevation gain, it is frequently hiked by more than 100 people on a nice summer day. But even with the physical challenge and the lack of solitude, this is still a must-do hike; those crowds of hikers know that the views here are truly superb. Stunning vistas extend for more than 100 miles, so you can pull out the maps and pick out landmarks for hours. There is also plenty of wildlife in the area, which may or may not be a good thing because the mountain goats here are sometimes a real danger to people. Call ahead about the latest conditions.

Best Time

The trail is usually open July–October. Though it's attractive any time that it is open, the trail is at its best in mid- to late July when there is still snow streaking the nearby peaks and the alpine wildflowers are blooming. Save this hike for a clear day (to enjoy the view) and try to visit on a weekday (to reduce the crowds).

Finding the Trail

Leave US 101 near milepost 331.7 at the north end of the community of Hoodsport. Turn west on

TRAIL USE
Day hiking,
dogs allowed

LENGTH
3.4 miles, 3 hours

CUMULATIVE ELEVATION
2,350'

DIFFICULTY
- 1 2 3 **4** 5 +

TRAIL TYPE
Out-and-back

SURFACE TYPE
Dirt

CONTOUR MAP
Custom Correct *Mount Skokomish–Lake Cushman* or Green Trails *Mt Steel* #167

START & END
N47° 30.615'
W123° 14.879'

FEATURES
High viewpoint, wildlife

FACILITIES
Restrooms

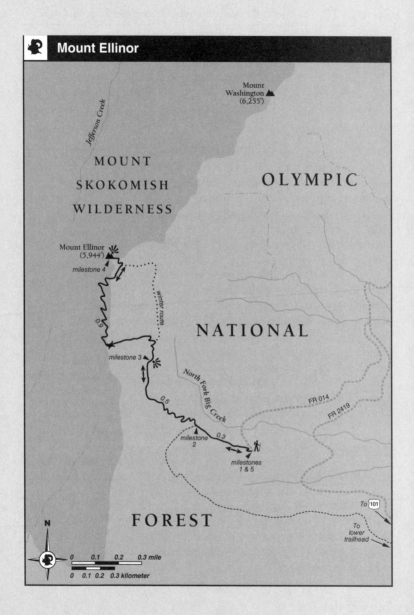

Mount
Washington
(6,255')

Jefferson Creek

MOUNT

SKOKOMISH

WILDERNESS

OLYMPIC

Mount Ellinor
(5,944')
milestone 4

winter route

0.9

NATIONAL

milestone 3

North Fork Big Creek

0.5

FR 014

FR 2419

milestone
2

0.3

milestones
1 & 5

To 101

FOREST

To
lower
trailhead

N

0   0.1   0.2   0.3 mile

0   0.1 0.2 0.3 kilometer

Washington Highway 119, following signs to Lake Cushman, and drive 9.5 miles on this paved road to a T-junction. Turn right on Forest Road 24, a good gravel thoroughfare, and proceed 1.6 miles to a junction. Turn left on FR 2419, following signs to Jefferson Pass and Mount Ellinor, and drive 4.7 miles to the lower trailhead. You can begin your hike here (adding 900 feet and 3 miles round-trip to your journey), but most people prefer to start at the upper trailhead. To reach it, continue driving on FR 2419 for another 1.7 miles, and then turn left on FR 014 and go 1 mile on this bumpy but decent route to the road-end trailhead in an old clear-cut.

Trail Description

Starting from the northwest corner of the small parking area, ▶1 the trail makes two quick switchbacks to a trail register at the top of the old clear-cut. From here, you ascend along the top of a ridge through attractive but viewless forest. At 0.3 mile is a junction ▶2 with the trail coming up from the lower trailhead.

You bear right at this junction and continue uphill, steadily switchbacking through forest and passing occasional log benches where you can sit and rest. The trail is often quite steep, but frequent log and stone steps have been installed to keep the

 Steep

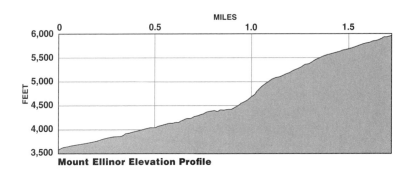

Mount Ellinor Elevation Profile

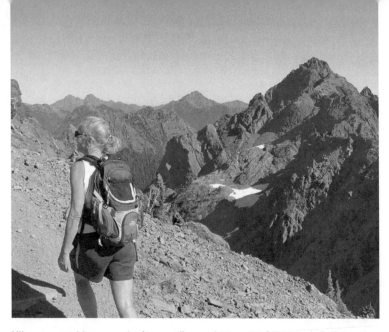

Hiker approaching summit *of Mount Ellinor with Mount Washington in the background*

Viewpoint 👀

grade reasonable. At about 0.5 mile from the junction, you pass the first good viewpoint, ▶3 which sits on a little rocky outcrop on your right. This overlook offers fine views of Hood Canal, a portion of Lake Cushman, and the towering distant mass of Mount Rainier.

Steep 🚶

From this point, the trail begins a steep and unrelenting uphill on a mostly open and rocky slope. This uphill continues all the way to the summit, and it can be a tiring ascent, especially on a hot summer day.

You soon pass a sketchy trail that goes to the right toward a rocky gully. This is the "winter" route to the summit, where climbers ascend a snow-filled gully in the off-season. Summer hikers keep left on the main trail and make a steep uphill traverse of a rocky slope to a little saddle on the side of the mountain. From here, you keep going steeply uphill, though your sweat is compensated by views that continue to improve with each tiring step.

Finally, at 1.7 miles (but, more important, after gaining more than 2,300 feet of hard-won elevation) you reach the top. ▶4 Magnificent 360-degree views from this grandstand quite literally overpower you. To the east are numerous towering peaks of the distant Cascade Range. To the northwest is snowy Mount Olympus. Almost straight down to the southwest is Lake Cushman. And, of course, all around are seemingly an infinite number of peaks and ridges of the rugged Olympic Mountains. It is even possible to see your car parked at the upper trailhead a rather frighteningly long way down.

 Summit

 Viewpoint

Another famous (or infamous) feature of the summit area is the wildlife. Chipmunks are abundant, and they rely on their unquestionable cuteness to beg for handouts from hikers (please do not give in to their requests because it is not good for the animals to eat human food). The other common denizens of this high perch are mountain goats. These animals frequently have little fear of humans and traditionally have come very close to hikers. This makes for great photos but is unsafe for both goats and people. These animals are wild and unpredictable and come equipped with plenty of muscle and razor-sharp horns. A few years ago, a goat attacked and killed a hiker in a different part of the Olympic Mountains, so the danger is real. During the early summer of 2012, several goats aggressively approached hikers on Mount Ellinor, prompting the US Forest Service to close the trail to all users (well, all *human* users) for virtually the entire summer. Call ahead to make sure it is open when you want to hike it.

 Wildlife

Officials now encourage hikers to scare away any goats that come close by shouting and/or throwing rocks at the animals. This may seem harsh to animal lovers, and it is certainly counter to the usual rules about not disturbing wildlife. However, without such measures the goats would either have to be killed or the trail permanently closed to hikers, so please take this advice seriously.

Having had your fill of the view, and taken plenty of photographs, return to the trailhead ►5 the way you came. *Note:* Be particularly careful on the descent because the trail is steep, and there are several places with loose pebbles and rocks, making for dangerous footing.

🚶	**MILESTONES**	
►1	0.0	Take trail from upper parking lot (N47° 30.615' W123° 14.879')
►2	0.3	Junction with lower trail (N47° 30.685' W123° 15.173')
►3	0.8	First viewpoint (N47° 31.170' W123° 20.065')
►4	1.7	Summit of Mount Ellinor (N47° 31.292' W123° 15.4.879')
►5	3.4	Return to trailhead (N47° 30.615' W123° 14.879')

Staircase Rapids

The brawny North Fork Skokomish River churns through a deep canyon in the southeastern corner of Olympic National Park. Just beyond the end of the road, the river tumbles over a series of boisterous rapids and small waterfalls that are easily viewed on a short and mostly level path right along the river's banks. Add in a beautiful and lush forest and you have a hike that is both scenic and easy enough to be fun for everyone. Because long-distance views are not an attraction here, this is an ideal choice for a bit of exercise on a rainy or cloudy day.

Best Time

The trail is usually open all year and fun in any weather; it's a good hike for rainy or cloudy weather. The scenery is most impressive in the spring and early summer when water levels are high and the forest is bursting with new greenery.

Finding the Trail

Leave US 101 near milepost 331.7 at the north end of the community of Hoodsport. Turn west on Washington Highway 119, following signs to Lake Cushman, and drive 9.5 miles on this paved road to a T-junction. Turn left, go 1.7 miles to the end of pavement, and proceed on a pothole-filled gravel road along the shores of Lake Cushman for another 4.1 miles to the boundary of Olympic National Park, where the pavement resumes. Exactly 1 mile later you come to the end of the road, where there is a ranger station, picnic area, parking lot, and trailheads.

TRAIL USE
Day hiking, child-friendly

LENGTH
1.8 miles, 1 hour

CUMULATIVE ELEVATION
100'

DIFFICULTY
- **1** 2 3 4 5 +

TRAIL TYPE
Out-and-back

SURFACE TYPE
Gravel, dirt

CONTOUR MAP
Custom Correct *Mount Skokomish–Lake Cushman* or Green Trails *Mt Steel* #167

START & END
N47° 30.928'
W123° 19.774'

FEATURES
Numerous rapids and falls on a large river, rain forest scenery

FACILITIES
Restrooms, picnic area, ranger station, water

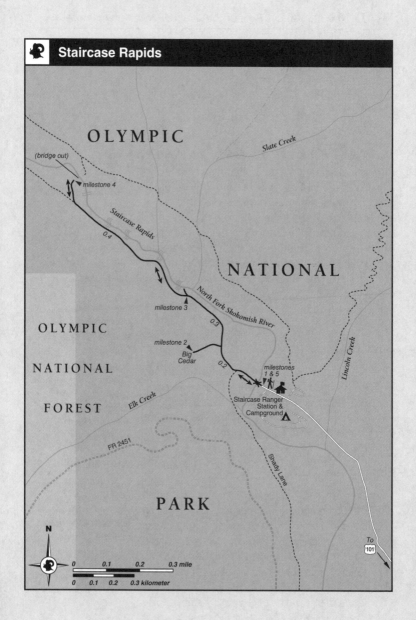

Staircase Rapids

OLYMPIC

Slate Creek

(bridge out)

▼ milestone 4

Staircase Rapids

0.4

NATIONAL

milestone 3

North Fork Skohomish River

0.3

OLYMPIC

milestone 2

Big Cedar

0.2

milestones 1 & 5

NATIONAL

Staircase Ranger Station & Campground

FOREST

Elk Creek

Lincoln Creek

FR 2451

Shady Lane

PARK

N

0   0.1   0.2   0.3 mile

0   0.1   0.2   0.3 kilometer

To 101

Trail Description

Several trails start from this location. For this hike, you begin at the northwest end of the large parking lot ►1 and cross an old road bridge spanning the North Fork Skokomish River. The large, rushing, and slightly turbid stream rumbles loudly beneath the bridge, giving you a taste of what is to come. On the other side of the bridge are a lawn area and a ranger's residence.

You bear right on a signed trail that begins just across from the residence building and follow a very wide gravel path beneath a canopy of firs, maples, and hemlocks. After just 40 yards, you ignore a possibly unsigned junction with Shady Lane Trail going left and continue walking the wide and nearly level main route. The trees here are huge and impressive and, along with the lush understory, create an intensely green landscape that is almost as vibrant as the dense rain forests of the Hoh, Queets, and Quinault Rivers. At about 0.15 mile, a signed side trail goes 0.1 mile to the left to visit Big Cedar, ►2 an almost unbelievably enormous giant that is now a downed log, but no less impressive for that. The diameter of the trunk of this dead monster is around 12 feet and stands about twice the height of even fairly tall visitors.

Old-Growth Forest

Back on the main trail, you continue hiking upstream past several very short side paths that lead to viewpoints just above the water. These paths used to be longer before the raging river pulled one of its all-too-frequent flooding fits and washed out the banks beneath the trails. A particularly excellent viewpoint comes at around 0.45 mile, where a path leads to a reddish-colored rocky outcrop ►3 that juts out into the river in the middle of a rushing rapid.

Viewpoint

About 0.1 mile after this viewpoint, you pass just above a frothing drop in the river that is sort of halfway between being a rapid and a full-fledged waterfall. In late spring, when the water is really

Waterfall

high, the noise emitted from this rapid is nearly deafening. Several more fast and furious rapids now come along in quick succession, giving appropriateness to the Staircase Rapids name. The last drop, truly a waterfall, is about 15 feet high and extremely impressive.

Just above this falls is a signed junction. The trail to the left continues upstream for another 1.2 miles to its end at Four Stream. This is a pretty hike, with nice forests along the way, but it is less dramatic than the Staircase Rapids section of the trail just described.

The trail to the right is labeled RAPIDS LOOP BRIDGE. That sign used to be accurate until floods wiped out the namesake bridge. It is still worth a short walk to the site of the former bridge, ►4 however, to marvel at the powerful river as it tumbles through chutes and skirts huge mossy boulders. Except, perhaps, in very late summer of exceptionally dry years, it is *far* too dangerous to attempt to ford the river, so please forget any such wild notions, turn around here, and return to the trailhead ►5 the way you came.

🚶	**MILESTONES**	
►1	0.0	Take trail from parking lot (N47° 30.928' W123° 19.774')
►2	0.2	Big Cedar (N47° 31.055' W123° 20.025')
►3	0.5	Rocky viewpoint (N47° 31.170' W123° 20.065')
►4	0.9	Washed-out bridge (N47° 31.452' W123° 20.528')
►5	1.8	Return to trailhead (N47° 30.928' W123° 19.774')

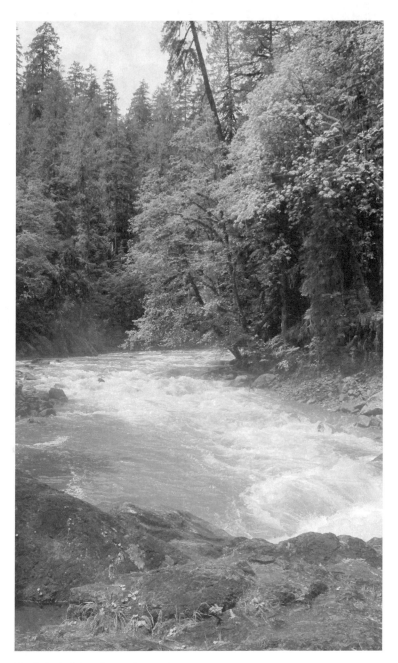

North Fork *Skokomish River from rocky viewpoint*

Appendix 1

Top-Rated Trails

As the title of this book implies, *all* of the trails in this book are great. Still, just like any athlete who makes it to the Olympics (the games, that is, not the mountains or the national park) is already among the best, he or she still competes further to see who is awarded the medals and is the best of the best. What follows are my selections for the medalists among these already great hikes.

Appendix 2

Governing Agencies and Nonprofit Organizations

Land Agencies

Olympic National Park

nps.gov/olym
600 E Park Ave.
Port Angeles, WA 98362
General Visitor Information: 360-565-3130
TTY (for the deaf): 800-833-6388
Road and Weather Hotline: 360-565-3131

Wilderness Information Centers (WIC):
Main WIC in Port Angeles: 360-565-3100
(Don't expect to reach an actual human being when you call—it almost never happens. Leave a message, and someone will call you back.)
Quinault WIC on Lake Quinault: 360-288-0232
Staircase Ranger Station near Hoodsport: 360-877-5569

Olympic National Forest

www.fs.usda.gov/olympic

Supervisor's Office
1835 Black Lake Blvd. SW
Olympia, WA 98512
360-956-2402

Hood Canal Ranger District
295142 US 101 S
PO Box 280
Quilcene, WA 98376
360-765-2200

Pacific Ranger District: Forks Office
437 Tillicum Ln.
Forks, WA 98331
360-374-6522

Pacific Ranger District: Quinault Office
353 S Shore Rd.
PO Box 9
Quinault, WA 98575
360-288-2525

Clallam County Parks
clallam.net/parks
223 E Fourth St., Ste. 7
Port Angeles, WA 98362
360-417-2291

Dungeness National Wildlife Refuge
fws.gov/washingtonmaritime/dungeness
360-457-8451

Makah Indian Reservation
makah.com
Makah Tribal Council
PO Box 115
Neah Bay, WA 98357
360-645-2201

Washington State Department of Natural Resources
Olympic Region
dnr.wa.gov
411 Tillicum Ln.
Forks, WA 98331
360-374-2800

Other Useful Resources

Road Conditions Information
wsdot.wa.gov/regions/olympic
800-695-7623

Snow Survey Information
tinyurl.com/nrcssnowsurvey

Tide Tables and Information
National Oceanic and Atmospheric Administration
www.tidesandcurrents.noaa.gov

Important Nonprofit and Hiking Groups

Friends of Olympic National Park
friendsonp.org
PO Box 2438
Port Angeles, WA 98362

Klahhane Club
klahhaneclub.org
PO Box 494
Port Angeles, WA 98362

New Dungeness Light Station Association
newdungenesslighthouse.com
PO Box 1283
Sequim, WA 98382
360-683-6638

North Olympic Land Trust
northolympiclandtrust.org
104 N Laurel St., Ste. 104
Port Angeles, WA 98362
360-417-1815

Olympia Mountaineers
olympiamountaineers.org

Washington Trails Association
wta.org
705 Second Ave., Ste. 300
Seattle, WA 98104
206-625-1367

Lodging

In Olympic National Park, there are several beautiful old lodges located at various points on the north and west sides of the park. Four of these—Lake Crescent Lodge, Lake Quinault Lodge, Log Cabin Resort, and Sol Duc Hot Springs Resort—are run by Aramark Parks and Destinations. Spending some time at any of these facilities is rewarded with excellent scenery and the opportunity to enjoy nature at a wonderfully relaxed pace. To learn more about these locations or to make reservations, call 888-896-3818 or check out the website at **olympicnationalparks.com/stay/lodging.aspx.**

If you are spending your time along the southern Olympic coast, then another old lodge on parkland, Kalaloch Lodge, is an excellent choice for the night. To contact the lodge staff, call 866-662-9928 or see the website at **thekalalochlodge.com.**

The largest city directly adjacent to Olympic National Park is Port Angeles on the north side of the peninsula. Here, you will find a full range of motels and other accommodations, as well as shopping, restaurants, automotive services, hiking supplies, and the like. The park headquarters is also located here.

A more limited range of motels and other services can be found in the somewhat smaller towns of Forks and Sequim. A *much* more limited number of services can be found in Quilcene, Hoodsport, and several other tiny communities that are scattered along US 101 as the highway circles around the peninsula.

Camping options abound in the national park (often crowded but very pleasant), on national forest land, at state and county parks, and on private lands. Depending on where you want to stay, you will find everything from modern campgrounds with RV hookups, showers, and the like to very primitive sites hidden deep in the forest with no amenities whatsoever. Similarly, the fees charged run the gamut from quite expensive to entirely free. On nice summer weekends, be sure to find a spot early in the day because the sites fill up quickly.

Index

About the Author

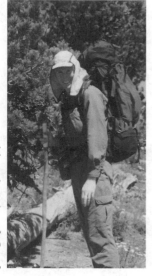

Douglas Lorain

Douglas Lorain's family moved to the Pacific Northwest in 1969, and he has been obsessively hitting the trails of his home region ever since. Over the years, he calculates that he has logged more than 33,000 trail miles in this corner of the country, including more than 1,000 doing (and redoing) the spectacular trails of the Olympic Peninsula. Despite a history that includes being shot at by a hunter, bitten by a rattlesnake, trapped in quicksand, charged by grizzly bears (twice!)—don't worry because none of these happened on the Olympic Peninsula—and donating countless gallons of blood to "invertebrate vampires," he happily sees no end in sight.

Series Creator

Joe Walowski conceived of the Top Trails series in 2003 and was series editor of the first three titles: *Top Trails Los Angeles, Top Trails San Francisco Bay Area,* and *Top Trails Lake Tahoe.* He lives in Seattle.